Children and Autism

Children and Autism

Stories of Triumph and Hope

Ennio Cipani, PhD

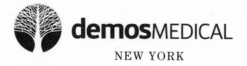

demosMEDICAL

NEW YORK

Acquisitions Editor: Noreen Henson

Cover Design: Steve Pisano

Compositor: S4Carlisle Publishing Services

Printer: Hamilton Printing Company

Visit our web site at www.demosmedpub.com

Medical information provided by Demos Health, in the absence of a visit with a healthcare professional, must be considered as an educational service only. This book is not designed to replace a physician's independent judgment about the appropriateness or risks of a procedure or therapy for a given patient. Our purpose is to provide you with information that will help you make your own healthcare decisions.

The information and opinions provided here are believed to be accurate and sound, based on the best judgment available to the authors, editors, and publisher, but readers who fail to consult appropriate health authorities assume the risk of any injuries. The publisher is not responsible for errors or omissions. The editors and publisher welcome any reader to report to the publisher any discrepancies or inaccuracies noticed.

Library of Congress Cataloging-in-Publication Data

Cipani, Ennio.
  Children and autism: stories of triumph and hope/Ennio Cipani.
      p. cm.
  Includes bibliographical references and index.
  ISBN 978-1-936303-01-4 (alk. paper)
  1. Autism in children——Case studies. 2. Behavior therapy for children.
I. Title.
  RJ506.A9C487 2011
  618.92′85882——dc22

2010031022

Special discounts on bulk quantities of Demos Health books are available to corporations, professional associations, pharmaceutical companies, health care organizations, and other qualifying groups. For details, please contact:

Special Sales Department
Demos Medical Publishing
11 W. 42nd Street
New York, NY 10036
Phone: 800–532–8663 or 212–683–0072
Fax: 212–941–7842
E-mail: rsantana@demosmedpub.com

Made in the United States of America

10 11 12 13   5 4 3 2 1

Contents

Introduction

Having a child show symptoms of autism can be both heartbreaking and scary for a parent. The deep-seated worry is that autism has for many years been a harbinger of a poor prognosis for living an independent life in mainstream society. However, it need not be so. There is now strong evidence to suggest that in some cases, with early intensive behavioral treatment (EIBT) over a lengthy period of time, their life can be vastly improved. This book presents the stories of seven children, diagnosed with autism, who received lengthy EIBT and their subsequent progress in school and life. In reading each of their stories, you will be amazed at their language, intellectual, and social development.

All seven children achieved what is referred to as "best outcome status" as a result of this treatment. Best outcome status is a child who does not present the symptoms of autism anymore. That is, they are indistinguishable from their same-age peers. You could observe them at home, school, work, or in the community and not see any of the signs or symptoms of autism. The current ages of these seven children are from elementary grade level all the way to a college graduate in economics (see "Chapter 3"). Their progress in skill development is documented by the behavior therapist who provided the services, taken from their case notes and data collection systems.

What Symptoms of Autism Are Addressed With EIBT?

Each of these seven children displayed severe learning and behavioral difficulties at the outset. Make no mistake; these children were diagnosed with autism but through EIBT, they began to exhibit behaviors that were age appropriate and socially appropriate. As you will read, some of the parents of the children in these stories were previously told by professionals to not expect much in the way of progress. It is fortunate that these parents did not give up hope but rather proceeded to find out how their child's lives could be improved. As a result, these dire predictions did not come true.

If you have a child with autism, you are probably familiar with the symptoms and problems that afflict children with this diagnosis. Children with autism display the following three major characteristics before the age of three[1]:

- A qualitative impairment in social interaction
- A qualitative impairment in communication
- Restricted repetitive and stereotyped patterns of behavior, interests, and activities

One of the most glaring issues with these children is their failure to develop appropriate social relations with others. For example, a parent may notice that their 6-month-old daughter does not smile back at them when they smile at her. They may also notice that their child does not seem to experience any joy, as other infants do when intrigued by something or someone. On the other hand, as a toddler, their son fails to take any interest in their presence and does not respond to his name by looking toward the speaker. As a young child, he does not interact with others, including adults, other children, and even his own siblings. Whereas nondisabled toddlers and young children show delight when seeing their parent after a brief time away from them and are delighted upon their return, such is not the case with parents of children with autism. Upon seeing their parent, the child may simply continue with his or her activity or fascination with an object he or she is engaged with. The child's response to his or her parents and others continues to be plagued with unemotional detachment throughout his or her early and middle development.

Nondisabled children take great joy in sharing events and activities with others, often saying such things as, "Look at___." Also, their attention to someone else who initiates such an attention-getting phrase immediately engages them. This has been referred to as joint attention and is noticeably absent in children with autism.

---

1 Taken from the *Diagnostic and Statistical Manual (DSM)-IV-TR*, APA, 2000, p. 75.

The good news is that an intensive form of early behavioral treatment has demonstrated that such detachment from the social world can be corrected in some cases[2]. As you will see in the following heartwarming seven stories, the children who received this treatment not only engage in age-appropriate social interactions with their parents but also have developed an important social network of friends and colleagues.

Leave me alone

Let us say that we have assembled a room full of preschool-aged children. As we observe these children, some are playing together. A few are playing by themselves, imagining that the toy blocks they put together form a castle for the king and queen. All of the children seem engrossed in their play activity except one child. This child is alone in the corner. He does not have a toy, book, or other item used in a play activity. Nevertheless, he is engaged in something. You watch him closely and you see he repetitively picks up the carpet corner (which is detached from the floor) and lets it fall to the terrazzo floor. When it hits the floor, it makes a sound like "plop." He is totally engrossed by the sound it makes. One child comes over to him and says, "What are you doing," in an inquisitive manner. He is unresponsive and continues to be intrigued by the action-reaction produced. Not getting any social response from this boy, the other child goes off and finds another child to play with. The boy in the corner continues the repetitive activity with the carpet for the entire play period.

During story time, this child does not seem interested in the colorful book or what the teacher is saying. He gets up multiple times and attempts to go back to the corner of the room where the carpet corner is unhinged from the flooring. He seems to be unnerved that the source of his entertainment during the morning is not available to him. The teacher's helpers bring him back to the circle area to be involved in the activity, but to no avail. While other children volunteer information about the story, this child seems oblivious to this activity and disinterested as well.

---

2 Although the overwhelming majority of the children in EIBT efforts improve a number of behaviors and gain skills in language, social, and pre-academic areas, only a certain percentage achieve best outcome status and become indistinguishable from their same-age peers, as in the case of these seven individuals in the book.

At the end of the school day, parents pick up their children. Almost every child is excited to see their mother and/or father and is verbose in the details of their escapades that morning. This joyous reunion is the case for all the children except this one child. When his mother comes in, he does not acknowledge her presence. Rather, he continues to play with the carpet corner. He seems oblivious to the ending of the preschool day. His mother calls him several times, but he does not even acknowledge such verbal requests, as if his hearing was temporarily impaired. She finally goes over to him and gets him to take her hand. He goes without comment.

A second prominent characteristic of children diagnosed with autism is a lack of language and communication skills. In some cases, vocal language is completely missing. They may use gestures and nonverbal behaviors when they see a rare need to communicate with others. In other cases, the child may be vocal but simply repeat specific words that he or she has heard. This manifestation of vocal behavior is termed "echolalia." Echolalia involves immediate simple reproduction of someone else's spoken language. Such children are unable to respond to simple questions such as, "What did you eat for breakfast this morning?" They will simply repeat the question, that is, "What did you eat for breakfast this morning?" with perfect imitative intonation.

Some children have delayed echolalia, where their vocal speech is simply an imitation of a phrase that they have heard previously, but is produced arbitrarily (wrong context, without any social function). Upon observation for a period of time, it becomes apparent that their vocal fluency does not translate to language competence. Such children might respond nonsensically to simple questions such as, "What did you eat for breakfast this morning?" with, "train goes down the tracks." If the child does have some basic language skills, it is often at a rudimentary level and certainly not at an age-appropriate conversational level. A child who is 8 years old may be able to identify three colors (red, orange, and yellow) instead of 30 different colors.

The seven children portrayed in this book now show usual or superb proficiency with the English language, in both social and academic settings. Their current language skills would not seem odd or deficient. Such a symptom of autism has disappeared in each of these seven cases. Further, their intellectual development has allowed them to proceed and succeed in life, both socially and educationally and in one case, in a demanding career.

Children with autism often engage in repetitive movements called stereotypic or self-stimulatory behavior. This repetitive pattern occurs to the exclusion of many other behaviors. If a teacher gets out a storybook with lots of pictures, many preschool children would immediately flock to the floor area, with excitement as they listen and watch. For many children with autism, their intrigue with their ritual pattern would take precedence over such a social activity.

What are some examples of stereotypic behavior? Some children engage in rocking in a chair back and forth over and over again hour upon hour in a single day. Other children engage in stereotypic behavior that involves flapping of one's hands repeatedly again possibly hundreds of times in an hour time frame. Such behaviors are pervasive over time, and it is often the reason why parents and teachers report being unable to "reach" children with autism. Although the children in these stories were initially plagued by a variety of such stereotypic behaviors, treatment produced dramatic results in this area. Two resulting phenomena from the children's treatment are very apparent: The seven children portrayed in this book do not currently exhibit such stereotypic behaviors, and they all have a diverse set of interests and skills in their repertoire.

Contributors

Audrey Gifford, MEd, BCBA, is a parent of a child who has, through ABA treatment, received a best outcome diagnosis from autism. Ms. Gifford has spent many years teaching both regular education and special education and received extensive specialized training in ABA and discrete trial training (DTT) as well as other behavioral methodologies. In 1998, she founded Bridges Behavioral Language Systems in the Sacramento, California, area to provide intensive ABA services to young children with autism. She lives in Citrus Heights, California, with her husband and the youngest three of their six children.

Tamlynn D. Graupner, MS, is cofounder and CEO of the Wisconsin Early Autism Project. Ms. Graupner is currently completing a doctoral program in Pediatric Neuropsychology and holds a BS in Psychology and Behavioral Science from the University of South Florida and an MS in early childhood development–early childhood administration from the University of Nebraska. Ms. Graupner's research interests include the study of brain differences in children with autism before and following intensive ABA therapy.

Justin Leaf, MA, is a graduate student at the University of Kansas who has worked in the field of autism for 6 years. Justin Leaf began his career working for Dr. Ron Leaf, Dr. Jon McEachin, and Dr. Mitchell Taubman at Autism Partnership, both as a behavior therapist and as a research coordinator. His research interests center on improving social skills for children with autism, developing friendships for children with autism, and comparing different teaching strategies. He is currently a private behavioral consultant in the Kansas City and Lawrence area, as well as the codirector of The Social Skills Group at the University of Kansas.

Ronald Leaf, PhD, is a licensed psychologist who has more than 35 years of experience in the field of autism. At the University of California, Los Angeles, he served as clinic supervisor, research psychologist, interim director of the Autism Project, and lecturer. He is the author of *Sense and Nonsense in the Behavioral Treatment of Autism and It's Time for School: Building Quality ABA Educational Programs* and coauthor of the book *A Work in Progress*. Dr. Leaf is a codirector of Autism Partnership. He is also the Executive Director of the Behavior Therapy and Learning Center, a mental health agency that consults with parents, care providers, and school personnel.

Jamison Dayharsh Leaf, MS, is a licensed marriage and family therapist. Ms. Leaf is the director of the Behavior Therapy and Learning Center. She began working with children with autism in the late 1970s at the University of California, Los Angeles, on the Young Autism Project, where she served as a senior therapist, research assistant, and teaching assistant. Ms. Leaf has worked with Dr. Leaf and Dr. McEachin at the Young Autism Project, the Behavior Therapy and Learning Center, Straight Talk, and the Autism Partnership. She has consulted on a national and international basis to families that have children with developmental disabilities. Ms. Leaf also coauthored *A Work in Progress*.

Rebecca P. F. MacDonald, PhD, BCBA, is a licensed psychologist in Massachusetts and a Board Certified Behavior Analyst (BCBA) who serves as the director of the Intensive Instructional Preschool Program for children with autism at The New England Center for Children. Dr. MacDonald has been at The New England Center for Children as the clinical director off and on since 1983. Dr. MacDonald has presented her research at numerous conferences over the past 20 years and published studies that have appeared in the *Journal of Applied Behavior Analysis*, *Research in Developmental Disabilities*, and *Behavioral Interventions*.

Glen O. Sallows, PhD, is cofounder and president of the Wisconsin Early Autism Project (WEAP). He has been working in the field of autism for more than 25 years. He received his doctorate in Clinical Psychology from the University of Oregon and trained with Dr. Ivar Lovaas at the University of California, Los Angeles, prior to starting the WEAP in 1993 with Tamlynn D. Graupner. Ms. Sallows and Graupner continue to study the effectiveness of ABA therapy and have brought this treatment to children in the United States, Great Britain, Canada, Central America, and Australia.

1

In the Beginning

As the saying goes, "we have come a long way." Autism as a separate and distinct disorder is a phenomenon of the last half century. The common diagnosis given to children who displayed the bizarre and unusual behaviors described above was that of childhood schizophrenia. In 1943 a psychiatrist, Dr. Leo Kanner, identified 19 children who exhibited characteristics and symptoms that he felt were qualitatively different than children diagnosed with childhood schizophrenia. He characterized these children's behavior by the presence of the following symptoms: (a) an extreme detachment from human relationships, (b) an excessive demand for requiring sameness (i.e., requiring the physical environment to be predictable), (c) an inability to use language to communicate, and (d) a fascination with objects. Based on his initial report along with a follow-up report of 120 children by Eisenberg and Kanner in 1956,[1] the identification of children with early infantile autism was founded. Perhaps the thing that most set these children apart was their detachment from their social environment. In particular, the child and its mother seemed to be unresponsive to each other during psychiatric consultations. It was probably this pattern of behavior that was a major factor in the formalization of this disorder and helps explain the theory that first emerged to explain the disorder.

Unfortunately, the child's unresponsive manner to their parents (and vice versa) led to misguided theories about why this would be. The term "emotional refrigerator" was coined in a book by a psychoanalytically

---

1 Eisenberg, L., & Kanner, L. (1956). Childhood schizophrenia. *American Journal of Orthopsychiatry, 26,* 556–566.

trained psychiatrist, Dr. Bruno Bettelheim, to describe the mothers of these children. His contention was that these children failed to develop appropriate attachment because of their mother's nonresponsiveness to their child. Although the phenomena he observed is a major feature of autism, it is fairly evident in current views that such behavior is not the result of the parent's emotional or behavioral response. Rather, it is the child's pattern of avoiding social interactions and not providing the social cues for attention, affection, and social reciprocity that is more likely the cause of the parent's lack of responsiveness.

As a result of this hypothesis, the cause of the child's autism was thought to be a result of the mother's emotional aloofness, and treatment involved psychotherapy for the mother. This prevailing (and ineffective[2]) psychoanalytic view dominated the field of autism throughout the 1950s and 1960s until two significant changes transpired. In the 1960s, the view that the disorder of autism probably resulted from neurological processes (and not the mother's response to her child) was advanced, chiefly by Dr. Bernard Rimland at the University of California, Los Angeles (UCLA).

The second, and I believe a more significant force, for examining autism in a different light was treatment research initiated in the mid-1960s providing positive proof that these children and their behavior could be changed. Dr. Ivar Lovaas, the founder of comprehensive early and intensive behavioral treatment (EIBT), developed the instructional procedures for teaching the basic building blocks of language and communication to children with autism. Many believe his greatest contribution to the field was his belief that children with autism could actually improve their language and social skills. In contrast to the other approaches at the time, treatment involved both the targeting of problem behavior and the building and development of language and social skills. The manner in which such skills were developed was called discrete trial training. His groundbreaking work with children with autism spanning a five-decade period demonstrated the profound effect EIBT would have on children.

Educational and language programs up until that time had not taken into account that some children would need thorough, regular,

---

2 Brown, J. L. (1960). Prognosis from presenting symptoms of pre-school children with atypical development. *American Journal of Orthopsychiatry, 30,* 382–390.

methodical instruction in acquiring the English language. The development of language was assumed to occur by the mere exposure of children to a language-enriched environment. Therefore, systematic teaching of skills that are requisites for more advanced language skills was deemed to be unnecessary. But that is not necessarily true. Even today, many preschool special education programs for children with autism are predicated on the exposure theory of language development[3] and that is not enough for children with autism.

Children with autism in Lovdas' nationally recognized treatment program were initially taught to imitate upon command, both nonverbal and verbal behaviors. Nonverbal imitation involved doing something, such as clapping your hands and having the child repeat that action. Vocal imitation initially involved making single sounds or phonemes and shaping approximations to those sounds. From these initial starts, the child was taught to come closer and closer to the sound being modeled until it was able to match that sound. From these early matched vocalizations, the child was then taught to imitate several words and then develop the skill to match any word produced by the therapist. After these children were able to imitate behavior and vocalizations, they were taught words to identify objects, actions, relations, and possession. Children continued working on these language skills, resulting in some of them speaking in short sentences after a time frame of a year.

Why did this effort succeed in developing language where other efforts had failed? First, in contrast to the psychoanalytic view, Lovaas and colleagues conceptualized the child's problems as one of skill deficit, requiring direct intervention. Providing psychotherapy to the mother had proved useless in terms of benefit to the child. Second, the EIBT approach was to directly teach such skills by presenting frequent opportunities to perform such behaviors until the child mastered them. The children were no longer expected to develop language from the natural course of play and interaction with other children and adults. Even today, this can be an issue in schools. Having children with autism who do not currently speak (or attend for that matter) in preschool activities such as circle time, story time, and so on, makes the

---

3 Exposure theory should be logically discounted and viewed as inherently flawed because children with autism often came from families where English is spoken regularly. This theory would only make sense in families where language is rarely used.

assumption that mere exposure will be sufficient for language to "take off." Unfortunately, for many children with autism, this does not work. The chapter "Why Artie Can't Learn" in this book addresses these issues in detail.

The results of Lovaas' initial work were published in 1973 in the *Journal of Applied Behavior Analysis*. It was the first report of empirically verified results from intensive behavioral treatment for a group of children with autism. Although the 1973 study demonstrated that the behavior of such children could be improved, the follow-up progress of the children in this first longitudinal project must have been disheartening. Although some of the children who went back to live with their parents maintained some or all of their gains, children who were discharged to institutions lost most if not all of the skills they acquired. Dr. Lovaas redoubled his efforts, insisting that treatment be rendered earlier in the life of the child and that it be extensive. Thus was born the EIBT model involving 40 hours per week of instructional training.

Lovaas' team continued their research on treatment for children with autism throughout the decades of the 1970s and 1980s, called the Young Autism Project. This monumental effort culminated in the landmark study published in 1987 in the *Journal of Clinical and Consulting Psychology*. In a nutshell, this research demonstrated that the use of EIBT for 40 hours a week delivered by well-trained therapists could produce astounding results. Nine of the 19 children receiving several years of 40 hours of therapy a week achieved best outcome status. As an example, the mean IQ level of these nine children was 109, placing them in the average range for ALL CHILDREN. Other available data on adaptive behavior, achievement, and school and personality measures indicated that the symptoms of autism have disappeared. They were considered indistinguishable from nondisabled, same-aged peers in their early elementary-grade classrooms (i.e., best outcome status). Only two of the 19 children failed to make substantial progress, continuing to have severe deficits and placement in special education classes for children with severe disabilities. This impressive display of the effectiveness of applied behavior analysis (ABA)–controlled empirical research is unmatched in the field of autism.

This finding was groundbreaking! Further, the progress of the children with best outcome status proved to be durable and resilient over time. A team of UCLA researchers published a 1993 follow-up study when these same nine children were between 10 and 16 years of age. They found that these children had maintained the "best outcome" status, that is, they were indistinguishable from same-aged peers in intellectual and educational functioning. These nine participants achieved such dramatic gains in language, social, and behavioral capabilities that they no longer evidenced symptoms of autism.

As a result of this study, in the late 1980s and 1990s, various regional centers in California, particularly the Central Valley area near Stockton Modesto and Sacramento, began implementing the intensive EIBT model developed by Dr. Lovaas. Today, EIBT in-home programs for children with autism are widespread, with some families in South Africa, China, and Europe implementing these instructional programs through behavioral consultants based in the United States. The real-life cases reported in this book are a testament to the research and treatment rendered at the UCLA in the last half of the 20th century.

2

What Is Applied Behavior Analysis?

If you have a child with autism, you may have heard the term ABA, which stands for *applied behavior analysis*, in connection with a treatment that is used with children with autism. Many people are confused by this term along with other similar terms, including early intensive behavioral treatment (EIBT). Is EIBT different from ABA? The answer is EIBT is a comprehensive approach that incorporates the principles of ABA. Applied behavior analysis can best be described as the application of a set of principles of learning and behavior that have been scientifically verified. Therefore, there may be variations of ABA, but all share some common characteristics.

You might be surprised to learn that ABA is not just for autism! The field of ABA has been involved in developing and subsequently testing treatments or interventions in a wide diversity of applied fields and human disorders. For example, principles of ABA have also been applied to children who acquire brain injury through trauma, people with health and obesity problems, adults with schizophrenia and other serious mental illnesses, problem behaviors in classrooms, instructional methods for teaching students from toddler age to adulthood (including college audiences), adult and childhood depression, as well as children with conduct problems and those diagnosed with attention deficit/hyperactivity disorder. There are even applications in the field of business, including the design of training programs, occupational safety programs, and performance management systems.

A common theme of ABA is the notion that people's behavior can be changed and that skills can be developed given the right technology. People who practice ABA look to the use of a science for changing behavior as the means to improve the quality of life. As you have just read, the development of EIBT at University of California, Los Angeles (UCLA) was predicated on the notion that these children could learn to acquire skills and that they were simply in need of a more advanced method of teaching them basic and advanced skills.

Guided by the belief that a scientific understanding of human behavior can improve the current status, practitioners of ABA are often optimistic about changing behavior where others feel compelled to accept the status as unalterable. It is often the case that parents are told their expectation is too unreasonable and that they should temper their efforts with the reality of the situation. Here is a perfect case example. I received a referral for a 14-year-old nonverbal child with severe disabilities who was expelled from school in the early 1990s because the school district claimed that they had tried everything to help him but to no avail. This child engaged in high rates of self-injury during instructional time. He had marks on his hand that showed physical evidence of his abuse to self, in the form of biting. The school contended that he could not profit from instruction because of his high rates of self-injury. In other words, they could not help him. The child's inability to profit from their instruction was his fault, due to his disorder, not the fault of their method of instruction. Try another way was not in their lexicon; hence, this child continued to have the same problems.

My behavioral specialist, Steve, worked with the child's father to develop an in-home ABA training program that would target two results: (a) decrease self-injury during task demands and (b) increase the number of tasks and activities he could perform without engaging in self-injury. How would Steve accomplish this? Our thought was that the child was biting himself due to his frustration over the type and manner in which his schoolwork was being presented. At school, this child was probably given assignments or instructional tasks that were far above his level of understanding. Further, if he completed a task, the result was the presentation of more assignments. In other words, finishing work meant you got more of it. This child's manner of escaping such a scenario involved self-injury at very intense levels. As a result, instruction and task demands probably ceased. We imagined that scenario replayed itself with daily regularity in the school setting. If he could talk, he might have said, "I don't know how to do this" or "How much of this do I have to do before I am done?"

We started by building a program where this child could currently perform without much difficulty. Therefore, Steve started with a small and simple task as the requirement to end the session. This hopefully would make the instruction more tolerable for this child and preclude any need for self-injury. For example, as soon as the child placed a block in the designated box, he was done. The child was allowed to leave that training session for a short earned break. After his earned break, he returned to perform the same task, with the same contingency in effect. As the child became very proficient at performing this simple task and earning time off from this task demand, the amount of work required was incrementally changed as a function of his performance. In one sentence, we achieved the following: You work (for a short period of time), and then you can do something more to your liking. This is a great life lesson for everyone to acquire!

Over a 1-year period of in-home treatment, two things happened. First, this child was able to perform a variety of tasks in training sessions lasting from 45 minutes to an hour. Second, he was not biting himself during these task requirements. In fact, during the training sessions at home, there were only two instances of biting. Remember, the school maintained that the child could not be educated because of his poor attention span and self-injury. They contended that such a state of affairs was uncorrectable. In fact, he was still biting himself at school during this same 1-year period. It is now obvious that the teaching methods that were used in the school provided a greater explanation for his behavior (or lack thereof). Remember, with consultation from Steve, the child's father became the teacher, using ABA. He did not hold any special teaching credentials or certificates. Perhaps what he did possess was the willingness to acquire effective skills and the love a father has for his son.

One might conclude at this point that the father had a special relationship with his son and that is the reason for the progress made. Steve and I would contend that if the training sessions had not incorporated several features including shorter session lengths in the beginning and contingent release from training via task completion, that the father would have probably generated the same types of opposition to work and self-injury as the school had. We firmly believed that it was the instructional strategy that produced the gains, which if replicated by others would have the same effect. The good news is that we were right; it was knowing how to teach this child was the difference maker. With the father's insistence (he threatened a lawsuit involving free and appropriate public education (FAPE)), the school hired a behavioral specialist to work with this child. Steve worked with the behavioral specialist to incorporate the home instructional strategy and a follow-up of school progress was done a few weeks after the child entered his new program. His father reported that he was doing fine.

What Can ABA Do for Children With Autism?

The original outcome research conducted at UCLA (and now at follow-up sites throughout the country) is the most impressive demonstration of the utility of ABA in the field of autism. There are numerous studies that demonstrate that individual skill deficits and/or problem behaviors or symptoms can be remedied through the application of ABA. These research studies have provided practitioners of ABA methods for addressing the variety of problems and symptoms of children with autism. Below are some ABA applications addressing the symptoms and problems of autism.

Spontaneous Expressions of Needs

If you have a child with autism, you may observe that he or she does not use language spontaneously, even though your child is capable of talking. For example, your child may be able to say "Apple" when she sees a picture of it, but then does not use her language when she wants an apple. For children who do not have autism, such a verbal expression of their needs and wants is a natural progression and is taken for granted. But for children with autism, the spontaneous use of their vocabulary can be absent, and their caregivers report that they have to be mind readers and anticipate their wants and desires.

Although some people may see this as an obstacle that is an inherent feature of these children, ABA personnel see it merely as a problem in need of a solution.[4] I and my former graduate students (who subsequently were teaching in their own classroom) often considered how we could get young children with severe disabilities and autism to express their wants and needs to adult personnel in the classroom. I believed that these children could develop such skills if the instructional and natural

---

4 Fortunately, there have been numerous research studies that have demonstrated that children with autism and other severe disabilities can acquire spontaneous requesting and protesting if the right strategy is in place.

environments were designed to facilitate such. However, it was going to require more than our just waiting around for the child to "mature."

In order to develop a protocol for classroom personnel that would facilitate spontaneous language in children with severe disabilities, I developed a program in the late 1980s that I termed, "the missing item format." The first phase of this program involved setting up an activity routine for the same period of time each day. We started with the morning snack, since it was already a daily routine in the classroom. During the morning snack, the children would be called to the snack table about the same time each morning. The snack items and utensils needed for the snack were set up ahead of time. Before the treatment program, the children merely had to sit down at the snack table and proceed to eat. In other words, language was not necessary to get food under this routine.

The students who were capable of labeling the snack items were ready for Phase II.[5] The classroom staff then implemented the missing item format. Before being called to the snack table, an item that was necessary for the routine to ensue was removed. For example, the teacher might set up the snack table to contain all the necessary ingredients except a spoon with which to eat the snack cereal. Removing an item such as the spoon threw a monkey wrench in the routine. The child would be unable to proceed until a request for the missing item was made. By engineering the environment to require some language response on the part of the student to obtain a spoon, spontaneous communication with an adult staff member eventually resulted over time.

As you can imagine, if the child was hungry, their motivation to obtain the spoon was pretty good. The delay in obtaining the spoon produced a condition under which language would become powerful. When the child said (or signed in some cases) the word "spoon," the staff person nearest him or her would respond, "Why yes I see you need a spoon, here you go" and proceed to give them a spoon. Of course, prompts to talk or sign were used in the beginning to get the child to initiate the request. The type of prompt used could be general such as, "Is there something you need?" to specific such as "spoon?" At some point (possibly over a period of days or a few weeks), the prompts were faded so that the child could request ahead of the

---

5 For students who did not yet expressively label any of the snack items or utensils, such training was provided apart from the snack activity and/or during the snack activity.

prompt and get the missing item quicker. With this approach, the child began to assert himself or herself and request the spoon upon seeing it being unavailable.

The missing item format was then used for other items of the snack routine. For example, the teacher might provide a cereal box, a container of milk, and a spoon and told she could eat her snack. When the child requested "bowl please" the bowl was immediately delivered and snack then ensued for that child. Across a number of missing items, these children eventually acquired the skill of "asserting" themselves when they needed something, a skill they lacked before this intervention. What was apparent to me and the other adults in the classroom is that children with autism could learn to communicate their needs. Further, anticipating their needs (and giving them what they desire without requiring language) was probably making them fail to develop such skill.

The missing item format was used as the initial strategy to develop the child's spontaneous language. However, with some children, language was only occurring when an adult faced the child. What was lacking in some of these children was the ability to get an adult's attention when one was not face to face with them. I did not see this as an impossibility. It just meant that I consider how the teaching environment could be altered to bring about the desired skill.

The program I developed involving appropriate attention getting began with a slight alteration of the existing conditions. The missing item format was still used, but the adult would not directly face the child during snack. Therefore, a request to an adult would require one extra step on the part of the child. I wanted the child to learn to tap the adult on the shoulder to get their attention. Conditional upon that behavior, the adult would then provide face-to-face attention and inquire what the child wanted. Then a request could be honored.

In order to accomplish the development of this added step, I told the adult to face away from the child but be within arm's distance of him or her. Prompts were used to get the child to tap the shoulder of the adult who was not facing him or her. When the child tapped the adult's shoulder, the adult would then face the child and emphatically say, "What do you want?" The child would then request the missing item, and of course, it would be delivered. As the child got better at getting an adult's attention at this distance, we now had to get the child to access attention irrespective of the distance between them and an adult. The adult was further away during snack so that the child would have get up from the seat and tap her shoulder. Naturally, with success, the distance between the adult and child was progressively increased.

This program was a huge success. It was not uncommon in this classroom for a child with disabilities to eventually learn to get up out of the seat, find one of the adults in the classroom, and tap them on the shoulder to get their attention, and then communicate their wants. When I watched this progression toward self-assertion, it was amazing to see these children begin to move on a continuum from dependence to self-reliance as a result of acquiring this pivotal skill. As you can see, ABA methods do not simply wait for the child to display the desired skill.[6] Our approach is to alter the environment so that the behavior you want to develop becomes more likely. However, at the heart of ABA practitioners is their belief that behavior can change and that children with autism can learn age-appropriate skills.

Look at That Mommy!

One of the phenomena that many parents take untold joy in with their children is the sharing of experiences. Having one's child show a great enthusiasm about their environment and wanting to share their observations with their parents and others seems to be a natural part of growth that does not need any direct intervention. For many kids, just an emphatic look from an adult or peer results in their attention to the item or event occurring. However, such is not the case with children with autism. Their interest in the environment and events surrounding them is often minimal. This is further compounded by their inexplicable lack of desire to share their experiences and interests with others. It is often the case that children with autism can seem oblivious to parental attempts to enter their world as they are enraptured by a random object of extreme fascination to them. Imagine what that feels like to a parent!

Teaching children to respond to another person's initiation of their experience in the social environment is called "joint attention responding." To reiterate, with most children, joint attention occurs readily. For an average 3-year-old, all one has to do is look and point

---

6 My department chair at the University of the Pacific, Dr. Hugh McBride had the following theorem "if you keep doing what you are doing, you'll keep getting what you are getting." I have used that logic over the years and thank him for imparting his wisdom.

at something in an excited fashion and the child will follow with their attention. Such is not the case with children with autism. They seem to be uninterested in the social events and experiences surrounding them. But again, these skills can be developed. ABA is about working to develop such a behavior when it is lacking so that these children can profit from the social experiences. What is apparent is that it just does not occur under usual conditions. Researchers and clinicians like Dr. Rebecca MacDonald have found unique and effective methods for developing joint attention. When the child with autism begins to take interest in what other people are excited about, they begin to learn from their social environment.

Getting children with autism to share *their* interests is also important. The development of "joint attention initiation" produces social development as the child begins to interact more with his or her social environment in meaningful ways. When children with autism learn to both initiate and respond with joint attention to the social environment, their world comes alive. The chapter in this book entitled "Look It's a Train" depicts such an approach to develop joint attention, both initiation and responding. Charts at the back of the book have some information on joint attention and the steps to developing this skill.

ABA and Destructive Behaviors

One of the most disconcerting problems that require behavioral treatment attention is a child who engages in severe destructive behavior. Some children with autism engage in destructive behavior that is perpetrated on themselves, called self-injurious behavior. When observing such behavior, it can seem unexplainable as to why they engage in such self-injury. These children will slap themselves in the face; hit themselves on the thigh, stomach, or other body parts with great force; bite themselves on the hand, arm, or other areas; and/or bang their head against the floor or wall. Most people upon observing such behaviors would be hard-pressed to find a reason for such behavior. In fact, several decades ago, this behavior was also attributed to the child's disorder by many professionals in the field. However, today we know as a result of ABA research, conducted by Dr. Brian Iwata of the University of Florida, that self-injury is driven by social context.

Self-injury is not as unpredictable as some think. For example, let us say that a child with autism plays with a piece string, moving it back and forth on the ground. The adult in the classroom comes to him and says, "It is time for our morning activity." She takes away the string and attempts to get him to stand up and come to the instructional activity. Instead of compliance, the child reacts violently as if he had suffered some physical injury. He cries and kicks his feet in the air as he falls to the ground. After a short interval of this incident, the child then slaps himself in the face. The adult not knowing what to do, and pressed to get the child to stop this self-destructive behavior, gives him back the string. This brings a cessation to this tantrum episode, whereupon the child happily returns to his ritual. Now, both parties are happy with this state of affairs. The child has his string and the adult has transformed chaos to peace. However, the long-term effect is that both parties have now ensured that when the child wants something, self-injury is more likely. When you view this analysis, self-injury is easier to understand. Self-injury is how this child gets what he wants.

I'll give you another example. A hypothetical 3-year-old child with autism, who lacks vocal language, wants cheese puffs. Until now, this child's crying has been successful in getting cheese puffs when he cries. Crying in this context is a very useful and adaptive behavior for this child. It has worked well in the past, although it might take a while to get what he wants. However, on one particular occasion, this child's mother is fairly busy and he has cried for over 20 minutes without apparent success at producing cheese puffs. The child is very upset, and he hits his leg. This brings his mother to him to investigate his frustration, and subsequently he gets cheese puffs to make him settle down. This is an unfortunate chain of events. The genesis of self-injury has now been seeded. Self-injury becomes more functional than crying in getting cheese puffs; therefore, the child resorts to self-injury more frequently. It also starts occurring earlier in the sequence of events. As you can see, this child has learned that physically abusing himself is very adaptive!

Self-injury also can be functional when a child is given a task demand. For students with autism and other severe disabilities, self-injury often has the effect of putting an end to an activity they don't want to be involved in. If this behavior occurs when the child is being taught, what do you think is being terminated as a result of the child's self-injury? You guessed it. The case where Steve, my behavioral specialist was providing consultation for the in-home treatment program would fit such an explanation. When the child engaged in self-injury at school, what do you think happened to him? We hypothe-sized that whatever instruction was being delivered at that time ceased until he stopped hitting himself.[7] Self-injury became this child's protest response of choice, and an effective one at that.

Got Attention!

One of the major issues with children with autism is their inability to profit from traditional teaching. If you have watched a teacher in a classroom, you might see her presenting a lecture, with most of the children attending to what she says and does. The ability of children to learn from listening and observing the teacher is the key to profiting from a traditional approach to delivering instruction. Unfortunately, children with autism often cannot acquire skills via observation. Their attention to what the teacher says and does is often nonexistent.

Many teachers of these children will often comment that they are unable to get the children's attention. Therefore, it becomes difficult for these children to acquire the skills they should from these teach-ing methods. Getting the child's attention is a prerequisite for them to learn.

To reiterate, the methods that many teachers are taught in their university training program just don't work with children with autism. The teaching method used has to ensure that the instructor has the child's attention. Here's a real-life example that depicts how exacting the strategy may have to be in order for success to be achieved.

In the early 1980s, I taught a unique class for future teachers at a development center for the disabled. This class allowed me to demonstrate how to implement basic instructional strategies with the graduate students in the special education program. Following con-sent from the parents, I usually worked with the children to achieve some level of attending to task before allowing the students to work with the child in a one-to-one instructional format. On a particular day, I was given a child who was to be taught to put 100 pegs in a pegboard independently. He had this goal for quite some time. It did not take long for me to surmise that it was going to be a long time before he acquired the skill unless the method of teaching changed.

---

7 For more information on understanding behavior, the reader is referred to the text, *Critical skills in decoding child behavior in the classroom* and can inquire at publishing@ecipani.com

Put simply, he looked neither at the peg nor at the pegboard when asked to complete the task. Rather, he would move his head about, looking at the ceiling, the wall, the floor, the adjacent desk, everywhere except the pegboard. Therefore, the teaching staff always physically moved his hand to pick up a peg. Then they physically moved his hand to place it in one of the empty holes, all the while he was looking everywhere else. In other words, he did not have to pay attention to what was going on. When he failed to focus on the task, the staff person just moved his hand accordingly until the peg landed in one of the open spots.

I proceeded by making several changes. I changed the task to a form board that had three shapes to be placed in the board. The shapes are much larger than the pegs thus making it easier for him to pick up the piece. Second, I understood that his attention and eye contact had to be established before I would help him. I was determined to get this student to focus his eye gaze on the materials and not the ceiling. However, I realized that repeating what had been done before would prove fruitless. Allowing the pegboard piece to be placed in its hole without establishing eye gaze to that movement was counterproductive.

Therefore, I first positioned the shape right next to the opening. I would hold his hand on the shape until he made eye contact with the shape. When he looked at the shape, I would then immediately and quickly move it into the hole, with his gaze on the process. Therefore, his gaze at the materials was a requisite for helping him move the piece into the hole. With this approach, that is, making movement contingent on eye gaze at the materials, his eye contact with the shape when I held his hand on it (and not moving it) became common. I had succeeded in getting him to attend to the task, if only for short periods of time at this point.

It was now time to require more focus on the process of moving the shape into the open hole. To accomplish this, I moved the circle further away from the hole, again requiring that he maintain continuous eye contact with the circle piece as it moved toward the open hole on the form board. With this progression, the length of time he had to focus on the task went from about 1 second of attention to several seconds of continuous focus. If he gazed at the ceiling before the circle was put on the hole, the process was stopped and we went back to the beginning. I did not want him to take his eyes off the process even for a split second! As you can imagine, this is a laborious process but the result was well worth the effort. This student learned to put all three forms, a circle, a triangle, and the square in the form board independently! Further, as he had to pay attention to the task to complete it, and he now had the basic rudiments of attention to task. My help was not needed. This would never have happened if the procedures to teach the skill had not been altered to require attention to task. Children with severe disabilities and autism can acquire skills, but one has to be willing to change the manner in which you teach them when they fail to learn.

Getting Sustained Performance

How does a parent or teacher get a child with autism motivated to engage in a task? Their interest in social interactions with people is minimal, and their interest in learning new skills is often not adequate. In the 1980s, ABA practitioners identified that these children's ritualistic behavior could be used to one's advantage to teach them.

In the early 1980s, I had a child who I was teaching at home. As it was with many of the children I was serving via in-home treatment programs, this child was mostly nonresponsive to his parents' requests. In one of my first home visits, I entered the living room and saw him bouncing on a small trampoline. I was there for about 10–15 minutes and noted that he had not stopped once. I decided to conduct an experiment. I went over and asked him to get off the trampoline and gently grabbed his hand and pulled him off the trampoline. There were a few common items that were on a coffee table a couple of feet away. I got his attention when I said, "look at me" and asked him to go and get the cup on the coffee table. To ensure that he knew which item to pick up, I pointed to the cup. He walked over to the coffee table and got the cup and placed it in my hand upon prompt. I provided praise, "very good you got me the cup thank you very much." I then motioned for him to get back on the trampoline. I then went back to the couch and watched while he bounced rhythmically on the trampoline. Five minutes later, I repeated the process and asked him to get another item on the coffee table. Again, to ensure that he knew which item to select, I gestured which item to select. He brought the other item to me. I praised his effort and allowed him to get back on the trampoline. Over time, I required him to comply with two directives in a single session event before accessing trampoline time. Thus was born my development of the instructional format I called the, *Get Me Game*. He was motivated to perform the task by the reward of getting to jump on the trampoline.[8]

The *Get Me Game* was used to develop instructional control with children with autism. It provided a mechanism whereby the child would engage in compliant behavior, by following a series of directives and then access a preferred activity. In the beginning, the selection of items is made easy by pointing the item out with a gesture, since the focus at this point is on developing compliance. In the case of the child mentioned above, access to the trampoline and jumping behavior was the result of his attending to a series of instructions complied with the request. Subsequent to its initial use with several children in developing attention instructional control, I began to use it to develop receptive and expressive language skills, as well as preacademic and academic skills (see Appendix B for the Parent Training Manual on the *Get Me Game*).

Some people might view this use of stereotypic behavior as a reward in the *Get Me Game* as exacerbating a problem symptom of autism. That it reinforces stereotypic behavior. However, we have often found it to be beneficial, when we allow access to such a treasured activity as a reward for following instructions delivered in the *Get Me Game*. Using stereotypic behavior in this way produces greater levels of compliance in the *Game*, and motivation to successfully complete the *Game* increases tremendously. The child begins to acquire skill through the playing of the *Game* and therefore tolerates lengthier instructional sessions of the *Game*. What also happens is that the rate and duration of stereotypic behavior during *Game* time decreases dramatically. In other words, as these children become more engrossed and *skilled* at the instruction being delivered, the need to entertain themselves (via stereotypic behavior and rituals) becomes less. It does not disappear completely, but it certainly becomes unlikely while we are trying to teach them something, and that is a good thing! The child is now open to learning from our teaching methods.

---

8 This arrangement between preferred (e.g., bouncing on the trampoline) and less preferred (e.g., getting items upon command) events was delineated by Dr. David Premack and is termed the Premack principle.

What Separates ABA From Other Approaches?

All the treatment approaches used with the seven best outcome children depicted in this book have many similarities in their characteristics. One of the defining characteristics of ABA is that its application with children with autism is built on scientific research. Contrast this with other approaches to treating autism that you may come across. It is unfortunate that there is not an agency like the U.S. Food and Drug Administration to regulate treatments for children with autism, as well as other childhood disorders. It is also unfortunate that there are still treatments proposed to the public that are based more on fantasy than fiction.

ABA has a five-decade history of research demonstrating the effectiveness of various interventions. There have been many studies showing that ABA procedures are very effective in treating the learning deficits and behavior problems since the 1960s. But even more important are the long-term studies done at UCLA under Dr. Lovaas that were published in 1987. To reiterate, his team demonstrated that an ABA program of 40 hours per week, involving intense instructional and behavioral treatment was extremely effective for most of the 19 participants who received such a program. He found that 17 of these 19 young children showed dramatic gains when compared to children who did not receive such intensive treatment (two control groups were used). In science, that comparison is significant in that it shows a cause-and-effect relationship between the treatment and the outcome result.

Contrast this amassing of research evidence with the prior approach to treating autism, that is, enter the parents into psychotherapy. No scientific controlled research evidence existed that such treatment was effective. The major support for providing psychotherapy to the parent, typically the mother, was based on psychoanalytic attachment theory. Fortunately, this theory has been disproven over time, as studies demonstrating that behavior can change in children with autism when behavioral procedures that were used became increasingly public.

A second prominent characteristic of ABA is that each intervention or treatment has to stand on its own. In other words, if it works for Charlie, but it doesn't work for Bob, then another approach for Bob is needed. I have often told students wanting to learn the trade of ABA that a master clinician allows their teaching repertoire to come under control of the child's progress and learning. If the child fails to learn with repeated practice under a given instructional plan, the ABA practitioner changes the manner in which the instruction is delivered. If the child learns, you keep repeating what you are doing to that point. The specific strategy or treatment is based on the individual child's response.

Given this requisite for each intervention effort to prove its worth, data collection and evaluation of treatment are of paramount importance. Unlike some other intervention efforts, ABA documents the progress of the child with respect to target behavioral and instructional objectives and goals. It is not simply enough to say that a child is getting better. Such was the case in a report produced from a psychoanalytic treatment program in the 1960s. The report simply said that the children "got better." Better in regards to what? Contrast this with the stories in this book. You will see that all the children's gains were verified by data collection.

Perhaps the most significant characteristic of people who utilize ABA is their belief that children with autism can make substantial gains and achieve "best outcome" status. This is contrary to what many other professionals feel, that autism and other childhood mental developmental disorders cannot be improved significantly. In fact, as some of the stories you are about to read will illustrate; parents are often told that they should learn to accept the shortcomings of their child. Too many educational and psychological interventions for these children often try to develop social environments that accommodate the problems of behaviors, rather than change the behavior. I believe that we must do better. We cannot wait for the development of a magic pill to cure autism before anything substantive can be done. Having a diagnosis of autism should not be a sentence of doom for the child's future. It is in this spirit that researchers, practitioners, and university educators in the field of ABA strive to increase the effectiveness of this technology for the benefit of all.

ABA Stories of Triumph

The primary thrust of this book is the telling of seven stories of triumph. Each of the children in this book was diagnosed with autism at an early age. As a result of extensive EIBT, all seven have reached best outcome status. Although they all are at different age levels, their presence in mainstream environments would not be viewed with suspicion by anyone. Each story has a different path to success, with various pitfalls that had to be overcome. But all share two things: ABA served as the mechanism for the significant change in their development, and they all reached a level of progress where they are indistinguishable from their same-aged peers. In some cases, these children have excelled in certain areas of development.

I hope you enjoy reading the following stories and observe how progress is achieved in an incremental fashion. It is unfortunate that there is no immediate cure for autism; however, the field of ABA has provided hope where previously parents felt dismay and doom for the prognosis of the children. This book should show you that behavior can change. However, behavior change requires a carpenter with the right tools. One cannot simply pick up any tool and hope that success will be achieved. With the right tools, a child's behavior can be improved and some cases reach a level indicative of recovery. As a fellow parent, I urge you to become the best carpenter you can be.

3

Diamond in the Rough

AUDREY GIFFORD

Graduation ceremonies mark the commencement of the next stage of the life of each graduate. For college graduates, that usually means the beginning of truly adult responsibilities. Starting a career, moving to a new city, perhaps settling down and eventually starting a family are all very real possibilities for the new graduate. It is the time for each graduate to start to mold the mark he or she will make on the world. Most graduates have an overwhelming array of options to choose from for how and where they will live and work. Last spring, my daughter Lisa (not her real name) graduated from college.

Lisa was more than ready to take on the responsibilities of adult life. She never forgets an appointment or to send in a form on time. She makes sure that everyone knows about family gatherings, even in our large family with several adult (and younger) children. She cares for her younger brother and sisters with competence and is a little overspoiling. She is frighteningly intelligent.

She worked her way through college with part-time jobs. She worked at Target for a while and also started her own side business buying and selling textbooks online and through thrift stores. This was so profitable she was able to buy herself a new (used) car while still in school. That replaced the very elderly Volvo she bought as a sophomore in college.

Lisa just started her new job—the one she really wanted, working for the State in a way that affects the environment. She has friends.

Audrey Gifford is both a parent of Lisa and a Board Certified Behavior Analyst.

She has an on-again, off-again relationship with a boyfriend, a fairly typical situation for a 22-year-old. She likes her new job and seems to get along with the people there. She is all grown up and on her own, and her younger sisters claimed her room long ago when she first left for college. And, like all mothers, I am shocked that she could possibly be so wise and grown up!

I would be proud of Lisa regardless of her history. But her success is all the more poignant, because 20 years ago she seemed to have no hope of a future like this. She was severely and (as far as anyone could predict at the time) permanently handicapped. I was told in no uncertain terms that she would never have a job, would never marry, and would live in a supported-living group home environment at best. I was told that my response to this news should be to enroll in a grief class to learn to accept the inevitable. At the time, I was very worried that she might never even be toilet trained by the time she grew up or that she would never be able to speak.

The Early Years

I never dreamed that a child with disabilities could be born into *my* family. Those children happened to other people—saintly types like the people in books and movies, certainly not to ordinary people like me. Lisa was born 2 years after her older brother. We lived in a suburban home in a small town, and I was thrilled to have two healthy children, a boy and a girl, exactly as planned.

A few months after Lisa was born, I began to worry that something was wrong. There were eerie incidents from the very beginning. As a tiny baby, Lisa seemed to sleep an awful lot. She never cried to be taken out of her crib in the mornings. Every day after I woke up, I went into her room, saw her contentedly sitting in the crib, and lifted her out. This was very different from the way her brother had woken up each morning. He was early, insistent, hungry, and loud! Lisa refused to sleep in our bed as a small child, something her brother wanted to do all the time. Even when her diaper had leaked and her own sheets were wet, she would leave our bed, go back to her crib, and stand there until I got up and changed her sheets. As a baby, when I put her down at night to sleep, she stayed very still. She was still in the same position I put her down when I came to get her in the morning. The covers had not moved. She was almost like a doll. She loved to be held, but only by me, and only in a certain position. She stiffened and seemed to be made of wood if held by anyone else or if I held her so that she faced me. She would happily spend all day seated (facing forward, away from me) on my lap in a rocking chair.

She was a very quiet baby. She never babbled. I did not know what her voice sounded like at all (except to cry) for many years. If given the chance, she rocked or stared into space. She stared at reflective surfaces such as mirrors and the blank television screen any time she was able to see them. (I was so frightened by this that she did not get a mirror in her bedroom until she was a teenager.) She never said "mama," "dada," or even that mainstay of toddlerhood—"Mine!" She seemed unaware that the rest of the world was worthy of her attention. She did not flinch at loud noises or cry when she stepped into scalding bathwater. She once stepped into bath water so warm it made her foot turn red, yet she never uttered a sound. She did not seem to be aware of what was beneath her feet. She calmly walked into a pool when she was around a year old and seemed surprised that she fell when she hit the water. A few months after that, she walked off the edge of a kitchen counter and hurt herself very badly. She put her teeth all the way through the skin beneath her lip and needed six stitches. She did not cry when she fell. She did not even cry while the six stitches were placed. Even the doctor that put in her stitches seemed a bit spooked by her apparent lack of concern. Many times I had serious doubts that she could feel pain at all. On the other hand, Lisa had frequent, very impressive tantrums about utterly ridiculous issues. She screamed inconsolably if her chair was moved from its usual spot or a little bit of ketchup was put on her plate.

Lisa did not imitate anyone else as an infant or toddler. She did not try to pretend to help with chores as other children do or try to copy her brother's play in any way. She spent her days lining dolls up on the windowsills and blocks along the edges of tables. She did not look at people, and if her head was turned toward someone she did not seem to focus. Early on I had thought she had wonderful eye contact because she seemed to stare at me when I nursed her. That changed as soon as she was weaned. She never played with any other children, including her brother. There are no pictures of her and her brother together as young children.

The potty training that had been accomplished so easily by her brother was a complete disaster for Lisa and was all the more painful because it fueled my ever-increasing suspicions. Most frightening of all,

Lisa often banged her head on the nearest hard surface, including cement floors and glass patio doors. She banged her head over and over, oblivious to anything else. Some days she did this several times a day. Other days she did not do it at all.

As Lisa grew older and her behavior became more bizarre, my suspicions grew impossible to ignore. At each pediatrician visit, I considered telling the doctor about my concerns, then decided to not mention them. I was hesitant to broach the subject with him, for fear he would consider me an overanxious mother, or, worse, that he would say I was right. Her pediatrician never asked me about her language.

Lisa was interested in things, not people. She hated all foods, especially chocolate and anything that had any "mushy" texture at all. That included ketchup, pudding, whipped cream, frosting, and especially soup. She hated all the foods her brother loved. (He saw this as a positive.) She loved to walk along the fence in the backyard. We did not realize it at the time but she was engaging in what is called "self-stimulatory" behavior. She was watching the streams of sunlight through the spaces between the boards in the fence.

Once we set up a picnic in the backyard. All of the things were ready on the backyard picnic table, even some foods she was likely to at least pick at. Lisa tantrummed every time she was carried out to her highchair at the backyard table. Finally we moved the table so that it was in sight of the dining table, moved Lisa's high chair back to the dining room, and had our picnic where I could see her through the glass doors while she ate alone in the dining room.

I found myself looking for ways to "prove" there was nothing wrong with Lisa. When she lined up the blocks, she often sorted them by colors—I told myself a child with mental retardation surely would not do that! It started to become difficult to see other young children in public—I often saw children younger and smaller than Lisa talking in the grocery store, and all I could do was look at my mute little girl and try not to cry. A younger little girl who lived down the street was playing outside one day, talking in sentences. Her mother was standing near her, and I asked, "Was that the baby talking?" The mother looked at me in surprise and said, "Well, yes, of course." That was the first time I picked up the phone to call the doctor; after holding it for a moment, I put it back down. I was not ready yet.

When Lisa was about 18 months old, she had her regularly scheduled DPT shot. I placed her on the couch when we came home. She did not seem uncomfortable; she just did not get up to walk anywhere.

This was not a problem until an hour went by. Then 2 hours, and more. By the next morning, Lisa still had not taken a step, and when we propped her up on her feet she simply fell over. We took her to the emergency room, where we were told she was simply reacting to the DPT shot. She never cried or seemed hurt. Three days after the shot, she started walking again as if the entire episode had never happened.

A friend of the family was a professional behavior analyst. He worked with handicapped children and adults. We sat on my couch one day watching Lisa bang her head on the floor. I asked him if we should be concerned about her development. He looked at me and would only say that if I was worried we should have her checked. That was another day when I picked up the phone to call the doctor. And put it back down.

One day, the neighbor with the young daughter came to visit. As usual, Lisa ran away from the front of the house when the visitors entered. As we visited, the small daughter played and talked to her mother. Lisa had, of course, rebuffed attempts to play with her. The mother was trying to get her young daughter to stop talking to the adults so much during the visit. The little girl talked incessantly, and it was hard for the mother to carry on a conversation with me. She looked at Lisa, sitting alone with the toys I had set out for her, and remarked, "She plays so well alone!" I even managed to smile at that.

As Lisa neared her second birthday, Christmas arrived. She was 23 months old and had still never said a word or indicated she understood anything that was said to her. On Christmas morning, we opened all her presents for her. She was not interested in any of them. Later that day, a family friend came over dressed as Santa. He was very gentle and soft-spoken with Lisa, but she resisted him and finally said "Go away!" I was ecstatic! Not only had she spoken, but she had put two words together! I rounded up all the family that were there for Christmas and asked—"Did you hear her? Did you hear her?!" She did not say another word for 9 months.

But, for a little while longer, I was able to convince myself that Lisa was okay. As 1987 arrived, I was unaware of all the changes that would be made that year, both in Lisa's life and in the lives of many children with autism. It was the year she was finally diagnosed, as well as the year that a seminal study was published that gave hope to the lives of these children and their families. All that spring I waited for her next words to come. We lived in almond country, and the almonds bloomed again, beautiful and bright in the springtime sky, but our world kept getting darker.

My suspicions continued to mount until the day I found myself becoming furious with Lisa when I told her to get in the car. Any other 2-year-old would have raced to the door, eager to go on an outing. Lisa sat on the floor, completely unresponsive to me. In disgust, I got in the car and backed into the driveway without her. When she still did not appear in the doorway, I stormed back into the house. Lisa was still sitting on the floor where I had left her, unaware and unconcerned that I had gone. By now I had become very angry and shouted at her. She did not seem to hear. I was far angrier than I should have been—after all, she had never come when called at any time before, so why should this time have been different? I was angry because at last I had to face the possibility that Lisa was not just stubborn, but that she truly could not understand what I wanted and did not care. I was terrified to call the doctor. I was embarrassed by my fears and afraid I would waste the pediatrician's time. I was afraid I might be reprimanded for not telling the pediatrician about my fears earlier. Mostly I was afraid I would be told I was right. Finally, that June, I made an appointment and kept it to see what was wrong with my child.

June 1987 (2 Years, 5 Months Old)

There was a Denver Developmental Screening chart on the wall at the pediatrician's office. Lisa was not able to do any of the skills it said she should be able to perform except the motor skills. The doctor examined Lisa and talked to me about what she could do. When I said she had never spoken, he said, "You mean *never!*?" He said she was significantly delayed—at least 8 to 10 months—and referred her for a hearing exam and to see a developmental specialist.

At last my long-standing, deep-seated suspicions had been confirmed, and, perversely, I refused to believe it. I told myself (and all my friends and family) that the screening was not very thorough. I told myself that a 10-month delay for a 2-year-old child was not really significant. I was not ready to deal with this information yet. An appointment was made to have Lisa's hearing checked. In the days while we waited for the hearing test, I often stood behind her, shaking keys and banging pots and pans. She responded sometimes. Other times she did not even flinch.

Lisa sometimes went to a local nursery school for day care while I worked for a few hours, 2 times a week. One day at school, an air conditioner apparently exploded, causing a very loud noise. One of the nursery school teachers came to me when I picked Lisa up to tell me that she was looking at Lisa when the explosion occurred. Lisa did not even flinch. I began to hope it was just a hearing problem. Much later, the nursery school teacher told me that Lisa spent a great deal of her time every day hiding in a "cubby"—a locker without a door—at nursery school. After a few months, the school asked to have her "stay home and mature for while."

I fought back tears as we received the results of the hearing exam. Lisa's hearing was perfect. There were only more dire explanations left for her delays. Over the summer, I started to try to get her to say a few words. Between June and September, Lisa spoke a total of about 20 words.

September 1987 (2 Years, 8 Months Old)

In September, Lisa was duly evaluated by Dr. Louise King at our local school district. Lisa spent most of the evaluation peeling the labels off of a box of 64 crayons. The official report noted that she could not be persuaded to perform imitative tasks. Most days she did not speak more than one or two words, if at all. The report issued later noted that exchanging a favorite object for a less favored one was "a challenge." It noted that Lisa responded more to gestures than to verbal requests and that imitative tasks could not be elicited. The examiner had considered the Stanford-Binet IQ test but decided that the Bayley Scales of Infant Development test was a better choice because it was more manipulative, even though Lisa was old for that test. During the test Lisa could not be enticed to imitate getting a toy with a stick, imitate stirring with a spoon, or imitate a crayon stroke. She did hold a crayon, put cubes in a cup, uncover a box, and turn the pages of a book. She was unable to name objects, follow directions with a doll, point to body parts, point to pictures, hand the examiner objects, or differentiate a scribble from a stroke. Her other test results were in the normal range in gross motor area only. The psychologist refused to discuss the test results with me at the evaluation session, and an appointment was made to discuss the results.

I dressed in my most professional manner for this meeting. I hoped it would make me less likely to break down and cry. I was ready to believe that the professionals were right and that something was seriously wrong with my child. We arrived at the school early and were ushered into an empty classroom being used for storage, where we were seated on very small yellow plastic chairs. Several other professionals arrived with the psychologist. Lisa's assessment results were explained to us in the gravest of terms. Your daughter, we were told, is seriously delayed in all areas. She will attend special schools and classes for her entire childhood. She will never read or write at more than a rudimentary "survival" level, and that only if she is very lucky. As an adult, she will probably live in a group home, though she may live semi-independently with an extensive support system if she receives intensive training. Her father asked, "Is there no hope, then?" The professionals replied that there was always hope. There was always the one in a million.

No one uttered the dreaded words "mental retardation" to us. That would come in a letter several weeks after the meeting. Their implication, however, was clear. I asked if Lisa could be autistic, because she could do very hard puzzles. They said of course not, that autism was a very rare condition. The "autistic" label would come from the doctors, but the school never did officially admit that Lisa was not mentally retarded. They insisted that she had an IQ in the high 50s and never changed that stance. When I presented my reasons to believe that she was more intelligent than that, I was treated as if my reasons were simply symptoms of denial of reality on my part. The report that came later (it was not presented at the meeting) was the first time I saw her test scores. Some were below the first percentile (see the table below).

SEPTEMBER 1987 RIPON UNIFIED SCHOOL DISTRICT TEST SCORES

Bayley Scales of Infant Development

Lisa was already 2 months above the upper limit for the Bayley at the time of testing (32 months of age)

Chronological age: 32 months
Mental development estimate: 17–19 months

Vineland Adaptive Behavior Scales

(at 32 months of age)

Communication: standard 62, age equivalent 13 months
Daily living: standard 70, age equivalent 19 months
Socialization: standard 61, age equivalent 11 months

Developmental Test of Visual Motor Integration

Less than 2 years 6 months (only score given)

I walked out of that meeting in a daze. There was nothing to be done immediately, though I would have given the world to be told there was something I could do to help Lisa. I know I took care of the children the rest of that day and the rest of the week, but I do not remember what I did. I did not even cry that day. That began on the weekend, when I had some time to think. The worst of the grief and anger and racking sobs came then and continued to some degree for many years. For a while I cried openly whenever I saw a child Lisa's age (or younger) talking and playing on a playground or at the store. It was a long time before I could stand to visit friends with "normal" children Lisa's age. It seemed to be forever before I could go an hour without thinking of Lisa's problems, and longer still before her problems lost their place in the center of my life. Every morning for at least a year, I woke up having forgotten. For a few blissful moments, life was as it used to be; then I would remember and all of it would come crashing down. I called my sister almost daily, simply to cry on the phone. She listened while she worked and was a great support to me.

After the meeting, Lisa was enrolled two mornings a week in a special education class for severely handicapped children under the age of 3 with mental retardation. There were no other options presented or available. In fact, that district was unusual in that it provided services of any kind for children under 3. The school people said that the class was an "enriched environment." Lisa came from an upper-middle-class home with two college-educated parents. How could the class be more enriched than what she already had? But I was shy and did not share my concerns.

The first day Lisa went to that class, I watched through a one-way mirror. All of the children were obviously severely mentally retarded. I cried as I watched her there. I was afraid that she would never learn there. She never did anything well in groups. Sometimes I watched, and, when she did not answer fast enough, her turn was skipped. One professional told me, "Learn to feel okay if she never learns." Another school professional told me that imitation could not be taught.

There were other heartbreaking moments. On the mornings Lisa went to the special class, the small yellow bus came to pick her up. The neighborhood children called this the "tard" bus. I was horrified several times by the appearance of the bus driver. Some drivers had biker tattoos (before tattoos were fashionable) and spoke barely coherent English. One time, the bus bringing her home was very late.

When the bus finally arrived, the driver presented me with a bag of cherries. The driver said she was late because she had stopped to go to the grocery store, *leaving the children on the bus in the parking lot*, on the way home. She seemed to have no problem with this idea. I resigned myself to driving the 40-minute trip each way.

On the whole, the people actually working at the school site seemed intelligent, upbeat, and cheerful. They accepted the children for what they were. They were acting in the best interests of the children to the best of their knowledge. They simply did not believe that anything could be done except palliative measures. They knew that these children were doomed to be severely handicapped for life. It was unlikely that any of them were aware yet of the seminal Lovaas study that had just been published, and even less likely that they would see that study as a reason to change their practices. (This is still a huge problem for many public schools.) Special education was the only place that welcomed these children. However, it was a permanent place for them, as well. There was no expectation that any of them would ever leave special education for a "normal" school or a normal life. It was important to me that the people who worked with Lisa believe she could learn. I felt as if I was always telling the school people that she could learn much more than they hoped for. She had great problem-solving skills, even though she could not talk.

I was the only person trying to provide any typical peers for Lisa. I felt she needed some children to learn from, because she was above the skill levels of the children in her classroom and none of them had the social skills she needed to learn. Educating children with handicaps alongside their typically developing peers was simply not done at that time. Children like Lisa were segregated from their typically developing peers at a very young age and generally never spent much time with them for the rest of their lives. They spent their childhood in special schools on segregated campuses with no typically developing children (as Lisa's class was) and passed their adult lives in group homes and, sometimes, sheltered workshops. In these places, only the supervisors were not handicapped. It was very rare to see people with mental challenges in the larger society. You did not see them in stores, at bus stops, or at restaurants, as you do today.

So I took Lisa to a different small nursery school in our town two mornings a week to give her that exposure to typical children. I told them she was "very shy" and hoped she would be allowed to stay.

Support in typical school environments using a trained aide was of course unheard of at that time. Even now there is rarely a systematic databased reinforcement and prompting system for children in these situations, but for Lisa it was a start.

October 20, 1987 (2 Years, 9 Months Old)

I loved October when I was growing up. The weather was finally tolerable, and, in a more innocent era, the days were still long enough to play a good while after supper until the streetlights came on. All the kids on our street would go to the school yard and swing as high as we could, seeing who could kick their shoes the farthest distance from the swing, and the real daredevils would even jump off. But never me—I was too much of a coward. October held all the promise of Christmas, and the tingling comfortable anticipation of the magic of that holiday. But 1987 was not a good October.

In October of 1987, Lisa was seen by a developmental pediatrician, Dr. Christel Cranston, at the Sacramento campus of the UC Davis Medical Center. This was decades before the MIND (Medical Investigation of Neurodevelopmental Disorders) Institute was founded there. Lisa's UC Davis evaluation noted very late speech, with her first word at 21 months and no other words until 27 months. She still did not imitate words, gestural games, or activities. The doctor noted that she was very good at puzzles. She displayed a preference for sameness. She still played only by herself. She sorted objects and lined them up. Her head banging was noted, as well as her staring, her not blinking when fingers were waved in front of her eyes, and her inconsistent response to sound. She had just had a battery of formal tests done by the school district, so no new testing was done, but the clinical evaluation was long and thorough.

At this visit Lisa was diagnosed with PDD-NOS (Pervasive Developmental Disorder, Not Otherwise Specified—an autistic spectrum disorder), as well as distortions in the development of basic psychological functions. At last I had a diagnosis I could agree with. Although she was now learning the names of objects, she did not use them in age-appropriate conversation. For example, if an airplane flew overhead she did not point it out to anyone and say "Airplane!" as a typical child would. She was now simply able to give the names of some objects when she was asked to do that, but still could not use verbs in a phrase.

Her learning was not fast enough to "make up" for the time that had past. She was falling further behind all the time. By now, I had started to have serious reservations that the special class was helping her develop at all, and, in fact, I was afraid that some of the things they wanted her to do (e.g., use sign language) were making her less normal.

I started keeping a journal around that time.

November 3, 1987 (2 years, 10 months old) journal entry

Yesterday I think Lisa pooped in the potty—a great step forward if she did, as she does everything else but eliminate in the potty process. I have my doubts though. I saw her pick poop up off the floor and put in the potty, then want praise. Frustrating.

Last week she put two words together! Can dress herself except shoes, some symbolic play (could be lining up) frequent tantrums when frustrated.

Haven't seen her bang her head in a while. Understands some directions but cannot tell how much comes from visual cues (When I get my purse she should get in car. When I point to garbage that means she should throw it away, etc.)

She loves cats.

Many of her words are backward tikitikat = kitty cat

Some days I hope.

What's happening to her brother?

Wish grad school was not looking so impossible right now

November 10, 1987 (2 years, 10 months old) journal entry

Says peek-a-boo ka cheeka chakoo

Inflection is right anyway.

I have taken her off Nutra-sweet—long shot but it won't hurt—very long shot. She stopped progressing around time she started stealing my soda. When I cut back, she improved. Will try. Anyway. Still NO success at toileting.

November 13, 1987 (2 years, 10 months old) journal entry

Another mystery poop in the potty but I think she dumped it out of her diaper.

She says thank you "dank oo." She still cannot touch her nose when asked. It's like a year was left out and she skipped all of the 2-year-old skills and started on the niceties before the basics are there.

Will she fill in the gaps?

A nurse from the state regional center suggested a Neurological Exam (EEG). I am thinking about it.

I sat for 10–20 minutes on the side of the bathtub every couple of hours waiting for Lisa to produce something while she sat on the potty for countless months. I felt as if my entire life revolved around taking her to the bathroom, and there had been no progress despite my efforts.

December 3 and 10, 1987 (2 Years, 11 Months Old)

Elsie Ratto-Joy, a speech therapist referred by Lisa's pediatrician, attempted to do a formal speech evaluation. Lisa was not able to complete the evaluation as she was not able to attend to the tasks well enough to obtain a score. The evaluator noted that Lisa seemed oblivious to spoken directions but sometimes responded a few minutes later. She had poor eye contact and was able to attend to tasks for only about 1 minute. She again was found to have significant delays in receptive and expressive language, as well as social skills. It was also noted that, after brief "training," Lisa could respond to "What do you want?" with two-word phrases (want. . . .) The speech therapist used *discrete trial* techniques during the "brief training," though at the time I was not able to recognize those. With this training, in only a few minutes she had taught Lisa something that she had not been able to learn in 3 months of special education classes.

December 18, 1987 (2 years, 11 months old) journal entry

Last month a behaviorist from the Regional Center came. She advised me to take away the diapers. Lisa finally started using the potty! She wets her pants only once every 3 or 4 days now. She is initiating sometimes and the end is in sight.

Later on I noted that the behaviorist did not tell me about ABA (applied behavior analysis). She may not have known about it at that time.

January 1988 (3 Years Old)

Lisa turned 3 years old in January 1988. I went to the University of the Pacific (UOP) and asked to audit some courses in special education. I was not at all sure that Lisa was benefiting from her special class with the children with mental retardation. I wanted to know how to truly evaluate programs for her so that I could see what should be happening for her at school. I explained my circumstances to

Dr. Ennio Cipani, who was the coordinator of the severely handicapped special education graduate department at UOP. He allowed me
to enroll as a student in his program. I was set to start in the fall.

February 23, 1988 (3 years, 1 month old) journal entry

Lisa can name things but still has no verbs. School wants her to do sign
language. I want that phased out. She can copy lines, circles, and crosses.
After 6 months of special ed, these are the highlights of her language
learning to date:

1. Sometimes (rarely) she will hand you an object if you name it.
2. She answered me once when I said "What do you want?" She said
    "Story!"

She is still so very far behind.

She continues to excel at puzzles, but everyone keeps telling me she
has mental retardation and that I need to stop being in denial about that.
(They did not change anything after receiving the UC Davis report.) I suppose there are worse things than having mental retardation.

I see some spontaneous speech now. Her teacher at special ed says
she "spaces out" a lot there.

What happens to her when we die? Will her brother have to take care
of her when we are gone? Can we do that to him? Could she maybe do a
make-work job at my mom's store?

She tested at 19 months in expressive language in speech. She can do
two words if they use the cards from speech.

Lisa's speech pathologist later cofounded an ABA program in the
Modesto, California, area. I believe she was using discrete trial techniques with Lisa even in 1988. Certainly Lisa responded more to this
approach (which we privately funded) than she did to any of the school
options. Lisa's speech therapy sessions were her only possible opportunity for discrete trial training. Speech therapy was only available to her
for an hour per week. That was not intensive enough for her to make up
her delays. She had not learned very much as an infant. She had to learn
faster than a normal child if she was going to catch up.

April 1988 (3 Years, 3 Months) Special Olympics

I understand there are children and families who benefit from participating in Special Olympics. But for Lisa and our family it was heartbreaking. Lisa's experience there illustrated some of the issues that we

faced and raised questions about some of the basic assumptions that adults often seem to make about children with special needs. All the children in Lisa's class were sent to a field trip one day to participate in Special Olympics. It was assumed that all of the children would do this, and the option of declining was not discussed. All the children were taken to the site on special school buses. Once at the site, the children were taken off the bus and herded over to a group of teenagers. They had never met the teenagers before. It appeared to me that the teenagers were there for the purpose of acquiring service hours or some sort of class credit.

All of the participants were handicapped. There were no typical children there, so all the children (including Lisa) were presented as disabled children to a huge group of total strangers. While I did not doubt that Lisa had a serious disability, I was not comfortable having this fact publicized in this manner. We lived in a small community. The volunteers and other adults there who saw Lisa would know that she was a participant. I was afraid that years down the road that would reflect on whether they allowed their own children to play with her or invite her to birthday parties or they would otherwise judge her before she had a chance to prove herself.

Not surprisingly, Lisa did not like being pulled along by the wrist by a totally unknown young girl. I did not think Lisa should be pulled along by the wrist, especially because she was pulling away and crying. When I approached to take Lisa to the designated activity, the teenager told me I was not allowed to be near Lisa. I was speechless and furious. Lisa's teacher saw that interaction and took Lisa herself to the activities.

The children were "motored through" various gymnastic types of activities. They had never done any of these things before and never would again. There was no indication that any of these preschoolers found anything rewarding about the experience. I believed that their crying was a loud and insistent indication that many of them (including Lisa) found the entire experience extremely unpleasant. Even the teacher looked embarrassed by the whole spectacle. Lisa simply panicked. It was an appalling experience all the way around. As far as I could tell, none of these 3- and 4-year-old toddlers with mental retardation had any idea what was going on. Many cried hysterically and seemed to find the entire experience an overwhelming, pointless nightmare. I took Lisa home after less than an hour.

August 1988 (3 Years, 7 Months Old)

In August, I started graduate school at the UOP. This was the first place I learned about the ABA therapy that has been repeatedly shown to be the most effective treatment for children with autism. In one of my classes, a videotape was shown of the "before and after" children that had been treated by Dr. Lovaas at UCLA. I was floored. These children had made huge gains.

Dr. Cipani allowed me to bring Lisa to a class that involved supervised "hands on" work with children with severe disabilities. All of the graduate students (including me) could work with her (and other children) using discrete trial training and other ABA techniques. In addition to discrete trial training, I learned about reinforcers, prompting, shaping, fading, and many more ABA techniques. The program Lisa was given seems very primitive compared to what my clients are given now, but for her it was enough. We saw huge gains, and I began to spend more and more time each day working with Lisa in this manner.

While all parents are teachers, we became language teachers and had the advantage of being able to provide an environment that reinforced (rewarded) language attempts to communicate 24 hours per day. I remember riding in the car running pronouns over and over. We would say "Point to your door, point to my door" over and over until she was able to do this, even out of order and with other requests in between.

I noted in my journal that one day the school used a reward system, though I do not think it was based on any specific criteria or data. The reward was always chocolate. Lisa had always hated chocolate. To this day, she still hates chocolate. Even as a fledgling graduate student, I could see that trying to motivate her with something she hated was not a good idea.

Lisa spent less and less time at her special class and more time with Dr. Cipani and me. She worked alongside his typically developing young daughter, Vanessa, as well. Even though Vanessa was a year younger than Lisa, we were often asked if Lisa was the younger, because of her delayed language and small stature. That was a painful question every time I heard it. I felt Lisa looked close to "normal" when she and Vanessa worked together. These questions were a reminder of just how far she still had to go.

October 27, 1988 (3 Years, 9 Months Old)

The school district was pressuring me to have Lisa spend more time in special education and no time at all with typical peers, even though I paid for that myself. We had asked our health insurance company to at least cover the costs of Lisa's speech therapy. The insurance company said that we could be covered for speech for her only if we could prove that it was helping. They said we had to take her to the Stanford autism clinic to see if she was improving. We made an appointment for January 1989.

October and November 1988
(3 Years, 9 and 10 Months Old)

At that time, we focused almost exclusively on language. Social skills were given less emphasis. Effective procedures to teach social skills (not just placing a child in an environment with a group of peers and hoping she will pick them up) were much less sophisticated than they are now, and Lisa had social issues that lasted at least into middle school. I often wish I had known then what I know now; many of these problems could have been addressed when she was still very young.

That fall, I noted that Lisa responded for the first time with compassion to another creature. The neighbor's cat had had kittens, and Lisa petted one in particular with gentleness and love. We had never seen her care so much for anything before. We asked the neighbor if we could buy the cat. He does not know it, but he could have named any price—I would have happily paid it! We taught prepositions, nouns, verbs, colors, shapes, and letter names. That spring we discovered that Lisa had taught herself to read! She picked up a book, *Love You Forever*, at a neighbor's house and proceeded to read almost the entire book on her own.

Once we discovered that Lisa could read, Dr. Cipani added a reading component to her vocal language drills.[9] She was shown pictures with the "S" made more obvious to teach plurals. There was a period of about 6–9 months when Lisa read with more skill than she spoke.

---

9 The use of text to teach vocal language when appropriate has been incorporated into many of our programs for several years now and is starting to appear more often in the peer-reviewed literature. At this time, however, it was fairly experimental.

Lisa was making very fast progress but was still a long way behind her typically developing peers. We took a trip to Disneyland over the Christmas holidays. Lisa became so upset at the Trip to the Moon ride that the operators had to stop the ride and let her off. Lisa and I went behind the ride and ran into a walking Mickey Mouse character. Lisa saw that and started to climb up my dress, with a new wave of terror. Mickey Mouse sat down on a bench, and we sat on the far end. He gradually and slowly reached out his hand, and after about 15 minutes she allowed him to touch the bench a few feet away from her without screaming.

As Lisa made progress with her ABA therapy, I became more critical of what she was doing in school. I insisted that keeping her in a classroom full of children with mental retardation and who had no language or social skills was not appropriate. The administrators offered what was supposed to be a class for communicatively handicapped children. Lisa attended for about a week, until I discovered that the entire class was deaf. They did not speak either.

I pulled her out of that class, and we began again searching for a better place for her. No one considered offering ABA for 40 hours per week and a typical preschool with support, as is now the standard for my clients. The ABA she received (including the discrete trial from speech) was all paid for out of our pocket.

December 1988 (3 Years, 11 Months Old)

At graduate school, I was learning about autism and other disorders. Lisa went to many classes with me. She was very quiet and just sat there (she had quiet stims) during the lectures. People often told me how lucky I was that she was so well behaved. I had learned to just smile and try not to look too pained by them.

A diagnosis of autism was still rare, and there was even less consensus about its etiology than there is now. One of the older theories about the causes of autism was that children became autistic because their mothers were cold and distant—they were called "refrigerator moms." One of the professors in one of my classes made that claim while I was present. When I argued that my oldest child did not have the disorder, in spite of the fact that I was the mother of both children, he said I must have parented Lisa differently for her to have developed the disease. That theory has now been widely discredited. At the time,

I remember sitting there with tears in my eyes, more than a little shocked that anyone could tell me to my face (and in front of a class) that I had somehow been so horribly cold and distant to my own child that I had caused this.

During December, I called UCLA to see if we could get some help from Dr. Lovaas. We were told the therapy would cost $50,000 a year, there were no openings, and we would have to move the entire family to Los Angeles. Also, Lisa was too old. Now I see my own clients not infrequently making enormous sacrifices to obtain therapy for their children. But, in 1988, I was astonished. I could not believe that such an effective therapy was not covered by our health insurance. It never occurred to us to ask the school district to provide it. Now that some districts and state regional centers provide these services, some families are able to help their children get the therapy they need when they could not pay for it otherwise. Although many families still must make great sacrifices because their local district or regional centers refuse to pay, at least some of these entities are starting to provide what the children need. Some families are able to access ABA through health insurance, but this is even more rare, even in the face of new laws that try to force insurance companies to help these children. In December 1988, there were no public funding options for ABA at all. We had another child to consider, and if we moved, there would be no income at all. We made barely more than $50,000 a year. We would have to find a way to do this on our own.

By this time, Lisa was working all the time. It seemed that during her every waking moment she was either in therapy or being "run" by me or one of the graduate students. Her day was filled with demands that she use language to request everything—"grunt and point" did not cut it. Once Lisa could name an item reliably, we insisted she ask with longer phrases ("Cookie, please"). When that phrase was solid, we insisted she ask with longer phrases still ("I want a cookie, please"). We learned to use specific praise ("Good talking!") instead of vague praise ("Good job!"). We learned that the normal sequence of developing skills is not written in stone. Lisa could identify every letter in the alphabet before she could differentiate between "yours" and "mine." She could read before she could use the past tense. She put together 100-piece puzzles before she could speak at all. We had to work with the skills she had to give her the ones she did not have. There was no "cookbook" or other prewritten manual to use, as simply mimicking the usual developmental learning sequence was not always appropriate for her. The only time she was not held to these standards was the two mornings a week she went to the special class the district provided.

Christmas day 1988 (3 years, 11 months old) journal entry

(evening of Christmas day) This year Lisa was finally able to open presents. She responded to some of the excitement of Christmas for the first time. She's still afraid of Santa Claus but she was better today. She spent a lot of the time running around in circles, stimming in mirrors, but at least she was excited and happy at Christmas instead of overwhelmed and scared.

January 17, 1989 (Almost 4 Years Old)

January 17 was the day of the Stockton, CA schoolyard massacre. If the Stanford appointment had not happened that day, Lisa would have gone to a speech appointment on the block where the massacre occurred, and at the same time. She was examined by Dr. Bryna Seigal and Dr. Roland Ciaranello. They noted diminished social referencing and said that she had just started to observe the play of other children. At this time she could play one interactive game with her brother. She did not show interest in her peers. By this time, she could greet the children who came to our house but then left them to play alone in her room. It was noted she could complete 40- to 80-piece puzzles. Some perseverative topics were also noted—day and night, sun and moon, and animal noises. Echolalia was noted. There was no spontaneous imitation of language, and she had poor topic maintenance. There was no turn taking. Her eye contact was poor and was even worse in interactive situations. She was still reversing pronouns and referred to herself in the third person. She lacked social responsiveness and social referencing. Some overly concrete imitation was noted—Lisa included an unnecessary gesture to reach the goal. It was observed that she solved puzzles by content (not just by shape). The doctors said this indicated higher level cognitive processing than is usually seen in an autistic child at this performance mental age.

The doctors' report expressed concerns about Lisa being in a special education class because all they taught were adaptive skills;

academic skills were not addressed. I was continuing to work on academics as well as language, and at the regular preschool she attended three afternoons a week she was at least exposed to colors, letters, and numbers in a group setting. On Lisa's Merrill Palmer testing, her score was 76 overall (4½-year level), but her verbal IQ was very delayed—at the 2½-year level.

The Stanford evaluation concluded that at the age of 2½, Lisa met the full criteria for autistic disorder. At that time, she showed a lack of awareness of others, abnormal comfort seeking, impaired initiation, abnormal nonverbal communication, absence of imaginative activity, abnormal prosody, abnormal speech, stereotyped body movements, and restricted range of interests. The doctors felt that she had improved since she was 2, and at the time of this evaluation she was diagnosed as PDD-NOS—part of the autism spectrum.

I was elated—at last someone official agreed that she was not mentally retarded! The school, however, ignored the recommendation. The special education teacher told me, "No one wants their kid to be the highest functioning one in the class."

February 1989 (4 Years, 1 Month Old)

Lisa came down with chicken pox while we were visiting her grandparents. She ran a high fever and developed the hallmark spots. Chickenpox was a very common disease at that time and was not considered serious in children. But Lisa was affected in very serious ways. She lost all the skills she had so recently developed. She became mute and unresponsive, lost her toilet training, and reverted to simply stimming all day. She started banging her head again, over and over. She remained like this even when the fever and spots had started to subside. I took her to the emergency room, and the doctors did not understand why I was panicked. A week after the spots had subsided, Lisa began to regain the skills she had lost, except for toilet training. It was many years before she could run a fever without throwing me into a complete panic.

Two months later, the doctor found chicken pox scars on Lisa's urethra. Lisa did not yet have the language to tell me it hurt. She had a minor surgical operation to correct this and regained her toileting skills after that.

Spring 1989 (4 Years, 2 Months Old)

We had given the special ed classroom with the children with mental retardation another try, but again I took Lisa out of that class. She was gaining speech by leaps and bounds, and I did not think she was gaining it in that class. She was far beyond the other kids, who also had no social skills. I had been told there was an option in Escalon, a nearby town, where the children were taught language and did not have mental retardation. After some argument with the district, the change was permitted, and she was allowed to switch to the new class. I had great hopes that at last she would be taught something at school that she did not already know. She had long since surpassed the level of the classes the district had offered her before. They kept insisting she had mental retardation. I felt my objections to what they were offering were interpreted as still more denial on my part.

The "individualization" the district claimed to be present in the classroom had consisted of minor and inconsequential changes inconsistently applied—one child might be given a different crayon or more help with a particular task, but all the children completed the same tasks every day. Most days I did not see even this level of individualization. All the children participated in the same group activities every day. "One-on-one" time was nonexistent.

Special education was a place children never left. Once placed, a child was doomed to be in special classes forever, until she "graduated" to special adult services and group homes. Regular education preschool was never provided by the district. Of course, neither was the ABA. Lisa's weekly schedule included two to three mornings of regular preschool, two mornings of special class, and graduate school (which Lisa often attended—she was given ABA there) with me three nights a week, as well as all day, every day, running drills in the car, at home, whenever and wherever she was, more or less constantly. We had nowhere near the sophistication we have now, but we had (barely) enough.

April 15, 1989 (4 years, 3 months) journal entry

Easter Sunday
   She has come such a long way!
   Just came back from [the friend who saw her banging her head when she was very young]. He says he never told me about Lisa because he

knew she had autism and was scared to tell me. Lisa has not been tested for a while. I hope to put her in regular kindergarten. I am afraid the school will say she cannot because she still officially has mental retardation. I think she will need a new IQ test to get them to let her in.

Some days I think she seems pretty close to normal, except that she tends to persevere on favored topics for months.

And there are other things:

She will not go to Christy's [the neighbor child's] house to play when I try to take her.

She has never been invited to a birthday party. No one in special ed invites kids to birthdays. And of course the regular ed kids would never invite her.

Six months ago [a mom of one of Lisa's brother's friends] casually mentioned that her son would have a big party and of course she would invite Lisa. I looked forward to that for months, but the invitation never came. I am sure that mom never knew why I was so frosty to her after that.

Other kids consider her babyish. They tolerate her and baby her. They do not invite her to their parties, though.

Lisa can sing lots of songs now. She can play interactive games with me. We've worked on that a lot.

She is still not good at picking up on subtle social cues—she only realizes kids are mad at her if they hit her.[10] She is always asking, "Is that silly?" She cannot tell without help. She still won't eat anything mushy except what has been run in trials.

June 1989 (4 Years, 5 Months)

Lisa's speech was tested again. Her one-word vocabulary was pretty good—she actually was in the average range! After so many scores that had been below the first percentile, that 53rd percentile looked like heaven! On another test (the SPELT-PRE), she was still below the first percentile. She had no plural nouns, present progressives, pronouns, past tense, linking verbs, present tense, or irregular past tense. Her receptive language was characterized by syntactic defects as well as pragmatic deficits. She was unable to track the referent in a sentence and did not shift to the conversational partner's model. She also had articulation issues. She was only 60% understandable in conversational speech (see the table on page 46).

---

10 The teaching of how to respond to social cues was still many years in the future for ABA programming.

JUNE 1989—TEST SCORES, MODESTO, CALIFORNIA (TEST ADMINISTERED BY SPEECH PATHOLOGIST)

Chronological age, 4 years, 4 months (52 months)

EOWPVT (Expressive One Word Picture Vocabulary Test)

Raw score: 47
Language age: 4 years, 7 months
Standard score: 101 (53rd percentile)

SICD (Sequenced Inventory of Communication Development)

Overall receptive communication age: 44 months

RECEPTIVE

Language age in months	Items correct	Items incorrect
40	84%	Directions involving plurals
44	89%	Identifying coins
48	67%	Speech/sound discrimination
48 +	50%	3-step commands

Overall expressive communication age: 40 months

EXPRESSIVE

Language age in months	Items correct	Items incorrect
36	75%	Regular plurals
40	70%	If-what questions
44	75%	Response to "how" questions
48	62%	Repetition of digits and words, using "how" questions
48 +	56%	Use of conjunctions serially

SPELT (Structured Photographic Expressive Language Test–Pre)

Raw score: 10 (below first percentile)

No use of or improper use of plural nouns, present progressives, pronouns, past tense, copula, present tense, or irregular past tense. Expressive language was characterized by syntactic defects as well as pragmatic deficits. Lisa was unable to track the referent in a sentence. She did not shift from the conversational partner's model to an appropriate response. For example, if the examiner's model was a plural pronoun and her response required a singular pronoun, she was unable to make that shift even though she used singular pronouns in her spontaneous speech.

Compton Phonological Assessment of Children

Lisa was 60% intelligible (understandable) in conversational speech. She was 75% intelligible with contextual cues.

September 1989 (4 years, 8 months) journal entry

Lisa can put 2–3 word sentences together and can put longer ones together if she is motivated. She refers to herself as Lisa but will say "I" for "I want." She reverses pronouns. She says things like hurt "me-self." She can do a lot with visual cues. She understands what, where, and possibly who questions. She knows all her body parts. She needs 10–20 seconds to process things sometimes and will often say "uh" to give herself time to think. She rarely repeats questions you ask her. She knows all colors and shapes. She can count to 12, and sometimes to 15. She recognizes most numbers but gets 6 and 9 mixed up. She is so good at puzzles! I don't know if she understands same or different, but she has been able to match for a long time.

She will not initiate conversation with anyone but me. She will not defend her place in line and gets overwhelmed in crowds and withdraws. She understands taking turns but rarely plays interactively. She will now display affection to a crying child.

She holds her crayons in a funny way.

She can cut with scissors but holds the scissors oddly as well.*

Can copy a +, 0, sometimes triangle, and once drew an A, but that may have been luck. She can make a face but has to be prompted or she'll color it in until it is unrecognizable.

She can eat independently but takes apart her sandwiches. She sometimes goes around the house frantically saying "go potty" until someone walks in the bathroom doorway with her. Other than that she is potty trained.

She dresses herself except for tying shoes, but she tends to dawdle. She does not like to wash her hands.

October 1989 (4 years, 9 months) journal entry

Saturday night Lisa put several sentences together for a questionable purpose—to throw a neighbor child out of the house. She did not touch her physically. I heard her say "girl out of my house, out of my house!" Lisa kept crying and would not talk about it—I was thrilled at all those words, if not the intent. I never did find out if it was justified. We have to do something about her social skills. . . .

---

* In 2007, Lisa related this story about her thoughts during her educational program in 1989: Bizarre—another memory—must have been September or October 1989—the rest of my special ed class was putting artwork together with precut leaves while I was cutting the leaves, but then I was cutting them too slowly so they gave me the precut leaves. I think it was the end of the day or something.

Thanksgiving 1989 (4 years, 10 months) journal entry

I have volunteered to be a Campfire leader (in all my copious spare time) so that I can get other kids to play with her. Also, they let boys join as well, so I have a way for her brother to actually get to spend some time with me, as well.

There was a problem at the special school. The teacher I had originally placed Lisa with had gone on maternity leave (twins) and they had a new person in there. I watched the new substitute teacher in the class. She did not let Lisa have the time she needed to answer the questions she asked. She did not call on her when she finally did raise her hand—that was a difficult skill Lisa had been working on a long time with us at home. She ignored her attempts to communicate. I did not talk to the teacher at all while I observed or afterward. Later that week the principal called and said I could not go into the class because I made the teacher nervous. She was afraid I would intimidate the substitute teacher. Once again, I pulled Lisa out of special ed. She was getting more from what I was doing with her anyway.

She is finally able to say something she wants for Christmas! She says she wants an elephant![11]

April 19, 1990 (5 years, 3 months) journal entry

I wonder if she dreams. Her father says he has seen her eyes move when she sleeps. She did not understand when we asked her if she dreams. She cannot describe them.

She cannot follow a TV plot. It is hard to even get her to watch something for more than 1–2 minutes in the first place.

It occurs to me that she can finally sleep aligned with the bed. She always slept in whatever position she found herself—horizontal, diagonal, whatever position she first lay down. Her covers are actually messed up now in the morning!

A friend said to me last weekend that when her son was put in regular ed he was way above average in academics but fell apart without one-to-one teaching. Now he is back in resource. Depressing, but I appreciate the warning.

April 26, 1990 (5 years, 3 months) journal entry

She is doing a lot better in her regular ed class than anywhere else except the one-on-one. Today a minibus came by to take her out of her regular preschool class to go to Special Olympics. Luckily I showed up

---

11 I combed through many stores that fall and finally found a toy elephant—we still have it.

as the bus got there, so she did not get on. The regular ed school had no idea why the bus wanted her, but they thought they had to let her go with them.

After all our efforts to get her to function in a normal environment, they would take her back! I am still furious!

May 25, 1990 (5 years, 4 months) journal entry

Lisa was taken for a follow-up visit to Stanford. Dr. Seigal saw no need for further special education except possibly in speech and language. We cried in the car a little. This was just as shocking as when she was first diagnosed. She is still perseverating, still wets her pants every week or two, still stims off mirrors, still won't eat mushy food, but at least one person thinks she is pretty close to normal!

Her reading is very good—better than her brother's at this age. She still has some mild hand stims—licking hand and blowing spit bubbles. She has a few minor eye stims as well.

Current perseverative topic: clothing sizes.

Dr. Siegel says watch for learning disabilities.

Lisa licked the closet mirrors right after we got home.

Oh well.

This July we go back to Maine to see my grandparents. Dr. Seigal says Lisa now responds to the outside world without contrived reinforcement and that she is past the threshold where she could still regress.[12] I sure hope she is right. I'm scared of being disappointed again. It will probably be a while before I dare consider her out of the woods.

June 1990 (5 Years, 5 Months)

Dr. Cipani did a new IQ test on Lisa that spring. I had asked him to do that so that we could get the district to allow her to attend a regular kindergarten. The district had already shown that it would ignore anything from the Stanford autism clinic in favor of its own tests. He tested her on the verbal portion only because that was her weakest area. In that test she obtained a score of 120.

---

12 Today the criteria for autism are measured with standardized tests, such as the ADOS, that had not been developed at that time. Had these been available then, I would not have considered Lisa's symptoms to have diminished to the point where she could be considered no longer handicapped. The social skills deficits were not seen as all that important in that era. While I do not believe that Lisa now meets any of the criteria for being handicapped, I also believe that she would have been considered as no longer meeting the criteria for any autistic spectrum disorder before the age of 6 or 7.

August 24, 1990 (5 years, 7 months) journal entry

Today the baby-sitter called me at work. Lisa threw up in the Mervyn's parking lot—went white as a sheet and looked like she'd faint. She had seemed fine before. Lisa stopped talking and would not let anyone touch her. No fever or headbanging or stiffening up. By that evening she was fine, though it was very scary when she would not let anyone touch her. She even ate soup!

August 1990 (5 years, 7 months) notes to present for IEP to enter kindergarten

Skills I wanted her to learn:

How to deal with the cafeteria and not let every child get in front of her. Her local public school offered kindergarten classes for the full school day.

How to compete with other kids for teacher attention in regular ed.

Specific incentives (reinforcement) for her to interact with other kids in games, taking turns, and so on.

Let her academics grow—teach them that she can excel at something—she spent so long testing below the first percentile that I have become a little nuts about proving that she does not have mental retardation. She is far above the academic level of her class—please teach her something new.

Please make sure she plays with kids outside at recess.

Please insist on her using full sentences, and please and thank you; she still has lots of reversed pronouns and problems with plurals.

Please do not look at her and say "uh huh" when you don't understand. After you do this, she quits talking.

As far as I know, none of those suggestions were ever implemented, but Lisa was allowed to attend regular education kindergarten with the teacher who had taught her brother. She was exited out of special education as she no longer showed enough delays to be eligible for it. It was almost the end of the greatest challenges for her.

September 13, 1990 (5 years, 9 months old) journal entry

[After a few weeks of kindergarten] I finally called her teacher today to see how she is doing. She says she was very pleased with Lisa. She was surprised she did not play much with the classmates she knew from down the street but has other friends. She participates and follows through directions and plays interactively in the classroom. She is not playing with other kids on the playground. She stays by herself at recess. No one seems to feel any need to prompt her or anyone else to play together.

She does not seem to need the one-on-one from me anymore.

January 1991 (Sixth Birthday)

Lisa was exited from the Valley Mountain Regional Center system as she was no longer eligible for services. The social worker told me she was going to look up exactly how to do that as it had never happened to any of her clients before.

April 13, 1991 (6 years, 2 months old) journal entry

Lisa was tested on the Woodcock Johnson last week. She is reading at the third-grade level (3.0), and her math is at second-grade level (2.0).

Not bad for a kindergarten child with mental retardation!

She is no longer as shy at school. She even plays with kids on playground.

When I asked about her past, she says, "I had extra help learning to talk because my brain did not work right. I used to be scared all the time." I said, "Why didn't you like hugs?" She said, "I didn't?" I shook my head no.

Lisa said, "No wonder I was scared all the time!"

June 1991 (6 Years, 4 Months)

Kindergarten graduation was a new phenomenon at that time. Lisa's brother had not done anything like it, so I had no idea how important it was. I had not planned to attend (it was at 10 A.M. on a work day), but once I got to work and told the other people there what was going on, they told me it was something I definitely did not want to miss.

So I arrived as the ceremony started. The children sang some songs and recited a few poems. The teacher made a little speech, and at the end the children all distributed pink carnations to their mothers. Lisa was indistinguishable from her peers, and as she handed me the flower I found myself crying.

It was a landmark day.

September 1991 (6 Years Old)

Lisa started first grade with all her classmates. She had not had an IEP for a year at that point. Her teacher did not talk to me much, but after a month I discovered that Lisa had been placed in the lowest reading group. She was placed in the lowest group for all the subjects that had groups. When I asked her teacher why, she did not give me an answer.

Lisa's friend from Campfire told me that her teacher treated Lisa like she was stupid. That was the last year Lisa attended a public school.

August 1992 (7 Years Old)

We moved to Lodi over the summer, and I enrolled Lisa in a private school. No one there knew of her history, and I was determined to make sure that they never did. I was convinced that her entire first-grade year had been wasted because the teacher had assumed she was still handicapped. I knew that these lowered expectations not only denied Lisa the chance to learn at an appropriate level but that they could start to convince Lisa herself that she could not learn. I needed her in an environment where she was not prejudged because of all the paperwork in her school files.

The new school asked for her cumulative folder that schools keep with the records on all children. Usually a child in second grade would have only a few report cards and perhaps an immunization record. Lisa's cumulative file was enormous. It was full of all of her special education files, including the ones the district ignored from Stanford. Cumulative files were available to teachers as a matter of course.

So when I asked for the cumulative file to give to the new school, I said I would hand-deliver it. On the way to the new school, I edited the file. All of the references to special education were taken out and filed at my house. The new school did not know about Lisa's history for 4 years, and then only in sixth grade, when she had a seizure in the classroom. By then, of course, she had long since proven herself to be an excellent student.

Lisa was very quiet at the beginning of the second-grade year in her new private school. The teacher considered her shy, but not out of the ordinary range. And in this school, without her history following her, she was invited to birthday parties, and children actually came to hers!

Third Grade (8 Years Old)

By third grade, Lisa had bloomed. She had a few real friends. A little girl from France was a favorite—perhaps they both knew what it was like to be in a foreign world. She liked to play teacher, and her class-room teacher encouraged this. Lisa still struggled with minor social

issues, but she was getting better. None of her teachers noted any difficulties. Lisa did not tell me about her problems with kids at school
until many years later. Lisa gradually improved her social skills
throughout her school years.

Summer 1995 (10 Years Old)

Around fifth grade, Lisa was part of a project done by the local FEAT
(Families for Early Autism Treatment) group to show what children
with autism could achieve. She was one of a group of children in a
swimming pool who spoke to the interviewer. The point of the tape
was to show that she was not distinguishable from her peers. Lisa and
some friends all happily participated—they did not need any excuse to
get into a pool!

Junior High

In junior high, Lisa had the usual troubles of an adolescent. She was
socially awkward and needed to learn to use vocabulary that was
"dumbed down" for an audience of her peers. At the time, I attributed
that to her extreme intelligence, rather than to her history of autism, but
of course the autism could have been at least a contributing factor. She
seemed to be involved in at least some unauthorized "toilet papering" of
neighborhood trees. I was never sure exactly what happened there, but
I hoped it was at least a social event. She once said she did not know
how to carry on a conversation on the phone for hours on end, the way
many of her peers did. I still do not have that skill either. . . .

High School

Lisa's high school years were a time of great social and academic
growth. She was in a wonderful all-girls' school. She was welcomed
and made true friends—at least one of whom she still sees. She had
her first romance. No one at the high school was aware of her history,
until one incident when she was hurt by a horse and had to see the
school counselor, and another time when a cover letter from a special
education packet from her preschool years mysteriously appeared in
her high school file.

She finally was given a mirror for her room.

In her senior year (2002–2003) Lisa faced the stresses all the seniors face about college. She had excellent grades and SAT scores—710 verbal, 720 math. She received many high school honors, including graduating summa cum laude and being a National Honor Society member and a California Scholarship Federation member for life. She was also the recipient of the Bank of America Science award. She had done a great deal of volunteer work with the homeless in soup kitchens and had helped me with my work with children with autism, as well. She applied to some very prestigious universities. None of them knew of her history. She was accepted to all of them except MIT, but even there she was interviewed. Among the schools that accepted her were UC Berkeley's College of Chemistry and Harvey Mudd. She chose Berkeley.

Lisa's high school graduation was a very formal affair. It took place at Memorial Auditorium in Sacramento. Each of the girls wore a long white gown and carried a red rose. The honors for each girl were listed both in the program and as she was walking to the podium. I knew that this ceremony would be an emotional milestone, so I thought I could adequately prepare myself. It had been a great many years since I had thought of Lisa as a handicapped person, but milestones like this were always a reminder of just how far she had come, and how close she had come to a lifetime of being handicapped.

But, despite my best efforts, I still cried at Lisa's graduation. From the time she was first diagnosed until the time she went to kindergarten, I had been convinced this day would never arrive and that we would have only the dreary prospect of a sheltered workshop or supported living services to look forward to at this time.

College Years

Lisa transferred from Berkeley after her freshman year and completed her degree at Sacramento State University. She did well at Sacramento State and graduated cum laude with honors from there, as well. In May 2006, she took the Graduate Record Exam (GRE) and obtained the following scores (200–800 scale): 690 verbal (96th percentile for GRE takers), 790 quantitative (90th percentile for GRE takers). She also scored 5.0 on a 1–6 scale in analytical writing. Her degree is in economics with a math minor. She had come a very long way from those endless scores below the first percentile.

During Lisa's college years, she wrote a letter to Dr. Cipani. She has agreed to allow me to share it:

From Lisa to Dr. Cipani

I'd like to thank you for helping me learn how to interact with the world. I was isolated and I became a part of the world. I learned how to play tag, annoy my brother, and ask for things. I later learned how to stand up for myself and figure out whether someone's likely to be lying. Now I am in college. I can always say I wished I'd learned the social stuff earlier rather than painfully later on, but you did the best you could and you knew how to enter my world. You didn't view me as some hopeless, worthless child unworthy of the help you knew I needed. You didn't assume that just because I did not learn to communicate through normal means, I was incapable of learning how to communicate, laugh, cry, love, work, and play.

Through your skill and patience, you helped me escape from the prison my mind had created. When I was incapable of communication, I could not learn about or understand other people. I suspect that most people did not understand me much better than I understood them. My world was probably just as foreign to them as yours was to me, especially back when few knew what autism was. By entering my world in ways I could understand, you helped guide me into the mainstream world, which has given me a chance to control my own destiny. I still haven't figured out what my goals in life are, but hopefully I'll figure that out. Even if I don't achieve all of my goals, I will have had a chance, which is all that anyone can ask for. It is more than I would have had without your intervention.

Spring 2007

When I was approached about this book project, I was asked if Lisa would contribute some of her thoughts. The following is from Lisa.

I don't remember much from before I could talk. The memories I do have are brief and disconnected from one another. I remember focusing intently on an object, such as a crayon or a piece of wire (you know Mom, those twisties you use for the garbage) and being able to focus intently on that item, to the exclusion of everything else. I remember thinking that people could read my mind, thinking that they knew exactly what I wanted. I can even remember hearing and understanding some words but not understanding that they were an attempt to communicate. Hearing a sound from an air conditioning vent means the air conditioner is on, but it does not mean the air conditioner wants to engage me socially. It was not that I did not care about what they said, but rather that I did not know that they were trying to say anything to me. I vaguely recall interpreting human words, from family and teachers alike, in a similar manner.

Due to ABA, I developed the language skills to speak and listen. With that foundation, I quickly developed the academic skills necessary to function in a regular school environment and more gradually developed the social and emotional coping skills needed to be a well-adjusted person. From 7th to 12th grade in particular, thanks in great part to peer and teacher support from the parochial schools I attended, I greatly improved my self-confidence and social skills. I have been working in a variety of part-time jobs since I graduated from high school, jobs ranging from cashier to tutor to online seller. I am about to graduate from college with an economics major and mathematics minor. I am still figuring out what I want to do with my life. There was a time when job interviews terrified me, but I have gradually improved my skill in that and other areas, and I know that I am not the only person who has ever been nervous at a job interview.

I have several friends, a couple of whom I talk to on a near-daily basis. I am thinking of either entering the workforce or joining AmeriCorps and then going on to graduate school. I consider myself a nerd because I like computer games and am in my campus math club, but not in a negative context. Am I still autistic? It depends how you define autism. By the time I was 5 years old, I no longer met the diagnostic criteria for autism or PDD. I was an odd child, but as I later improved my social skills and found peers whose interests aligned with mine, I grew into a well-adjusted adolescent and adult. Whatever physical issues caused the autism are still there, and I do still have to manage occasional bouts with insomnia. More important however, is the fact that I am generally well adjusted to my environment. My life is profoundly better than it would have been if I had not received effective intervention.

—Lisa

4

Maggie Mae

AUDREY GIFFORD

If I could paint, I would paint a picture of 6-year-old Maggie flying through the gray winter day on an enormous horse, with her hair blowing behind her as she urged her horse to speed across the fields. I would paint a picture of her looking at me with curiosity and wonder and childish open-mindedness. I would paint a picture of a school play, a medal on a ribbon. A little girl who puts a heart for the dot on the "i" in her name. A little girl whose favorite book (for the moment) is *My Friend Flicka*. A girl who organized the children in her rural neighborhood to present a funeral for a pet rabbit. I would paint a picture of a child with a future as bright as she cares to paint it.

Maggie wants to be a veterinarian when she grows up. She has already broken in her first pony, at the tender age of 6. Her mother hopes she will specialize in equine veterinary practice because she loves horses so much and there is a great demand for that kind of vet. No one seems worried about the academic rigors of this kind of study—Maggie does all her school work easily, quickly, and very well. She is a model student, noted for her empathy for friends and animals. She won a third-place medal for her performance at the school oral language fair. Her teacher and principal (who are unaware of her history) say she does very well at school. She is at the top of her class, even though she is one of the youngest children in the class. She is well liked by her classmates and is invited to many birthday parties, even those that do not include the entire class. No one doubts that once she sets her mind to it, Maggie will become whatever she wants to when she grows up.

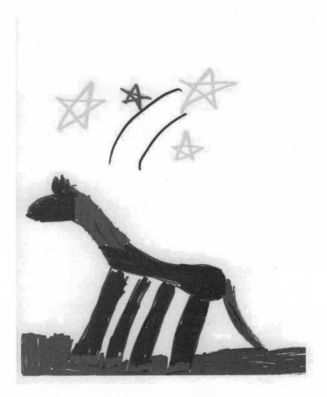

Maggie's artwork was used by her school as a greeting card.

Autism is something that Maggie's mother rarely thinks about in regard to Maggie any more, but at one time it was the defining factor of her entire life.

The Early Years

Maggie's mother remembers worrying about her speech as a small infant. She used very few words (and lost the ones she had at about 18 months) and repeated the same sound over and over. Her records show there were also repetitive behaviors and socially withdrawn behaviors at that age. Her lack of speech led her family to ask for an evaluation. This was done when Maggie was 29 months old by a psychologist from the Early Developmental Assessment and Diagnosis office via a referral from the local state agency (Alta California Regional Center).

Maggie's original diagnostic assessment noted echolalic speech (repeating the same words over and over) and little interest in other children, both in initiating attempts to play and in responding to attempts to play from another child. She did not engage in cooperative or parallel play with peers. A ritualized activity involving putting playing cards from a deck into adults' hands was observed. The psychologist noted that if Maggie was prevented from performing every step in an exact, predetermined order, she became very upset.

Maggie licked the surfaces of inedible objects, squeezed herself into tight places, and locked her gaze on objects while swiveling her head from side to side. She lined up crayons and other objects for hours if allowed to. She had once locked herself in a dark closet and showed no signs of alarm. The family found her asleep in the closet in the mornirg. She displayed no distress when injured. Her psychologist reported an incident in which Maggie remained passive and unconcerned when she had a thorn in her foot. She also seemed to have no reaction to another accident in which she burned her arm. She was noted to display some aggression toward other children.

Maggie was given standardized tests as part of that psychological assessment. Her scores were delayed in all areas except motor skills. The level of delay varied. Scores were significantly delayed in the auditory comprehension, daily living, and socialization domains. Scores were mildly delayed in the cognitive and expressive communication domain. Her age-equivalent scores (she was tested at 29 months of age) ranged from 13 months in the socialization domain to 21 months in the expressive communication domain. She met six of the criteria required for a diagnosis of autistic disorder (see the table on page 60). Her score on the Childhood Autism Rating Scale was 31, which placed her in the autism range. Maggie was given a diagnosis of autism on July 17, 2002, by Dr. Thomas Leigh. A separate diagnosis was also made by her Kaiser HMO physician. See the table on page 60 provides the details of this testing data.

Maggie's family was crushed. Her mother remembers that she thought Maggie would never be able to do anything. She would never get married or be independent. Maggie has older twin brothers, one with Asperger's syndrome and one with cerebral palsy. The challenges of parenting three small children with severe special needs would be formidable to anyone.

Maggie became a client of the Alta California Regional Center. The California Regional Center system serves people with developmental

MAGGIE'S PRESENTING SYMPTOMS THAT MET *DSM-IV* CRITERIA FOR AUTISTIC DISORDER

1. Marked impairments in the use of multiple nonverbal behaviors such as eye-to-eye gaze, facial expression, body postures, and gestures to regulate social interaction
2. Failure to develop peer relationships appropriate to developmental level
3. A lack of spontaneous seeking to share enjoyment, interests, or achievements with other people (e.g., by a lack of showing, bringing, or pointing out objects of interest to other people)
4. Delay in or total lack of, the development of spoken language (not accompanied by an attempt to compensate through alternative modes of communication such as gesture or mime)
5. Lack of varied, spontaneous make-believe play or social imitative play appropriate to developmental level
6. Encompassing preoccupation with one or more stereotyped and restricted patterns of interest that is abnormal either in intensity or focus

TESTING DATA FOR MAGGIE

Developmental Domain	Standard Score	Age Equivalent (Months)	Test Name
Cognitive	83	18	DAYC
Auditory comprehension	67	15	PLS-4
Expressive communication	83	21	PLS-4
Daily living skills	67	17	VABS
Socialization	68	13	VABS
Motor skills	99	29	VABS

DAYC (Developmental Assessment of Young Children—Cognitive Subtest)
PLS-4 (Preschool Language Scale—4th Edition)
VABS (Vineland Adaptive Behavior Scales—Interview Edition, Expanded Form)

disabilities such as retardation and autism. At some point after the original diagnosis, Maggie's parents learned about ABA (Applied Behavior Analysis) therapy. They had not been aware of this option for their child. The psychologist had recommended a functional skills "behavior analytic intervention" until Maggie turned 3, at which time he recommended that she be placed in a special education classroom. Once the family learned about ABA therapy, they contacted the Regional Center with a request for an ABA assessment and chose Bridges to provide that assessment and her ABA program. Her progress was described in detail over the course of her treatment.

October 2002 (Initial Assessment)

Maggie came to us for her assessment very young (30 months). She was tiny for her age, and her food intolerances had left her very thin. She was seriously underweight and had several health issues for much of the time we worked with her. At that time, Maggie had no way to ask for the things she needed and very few play skills. She had frequent severe tantrums every time the routine of her life was altered or when simple demands were placed on her, such as when she was asked to eat at a table or have her hair washed. Her initial referral notes that she was afraid of baby dolls and unfamiliar men. At the time she was assessed, she played appropriately for an average of 45 seconds before engaging in self-stimulatory behaviors (repetitively lining toys up or putting toys together in matched sets). Maggie was able to speak to some degree but did not use her language to interact with others or to ask for things she wanted. She was observed engaging in echolalia and other self-stimulatory behaviors.

During the assessment, Maggie sometimes screamed or acted fearful when given a task. She had several inappropriate behaviors that needed to be addressed, in addition to the echolalia. These included purposely spilling liquids and food on herself and lying down on the ground to allow the family dogs to lick her body. Her parents stated that they were most concerned about Maggie's aggression toward others, tantrumming, and self-stimulatory behaviors.

After reviewing the data from Maggie's initial assessment, we prescribed 25 hours per week of ABA programing. The low number was because of Maggie's need for naps and her very young age. Additionally, Maggie was prescribed 5 hours per month of direct supervision by a program director with a master's degree and several years of experience, as well as 15 hours per month of supervision by a consultant with a bachelor's degree and several years of experience. Her program was implemented 52 weeks a year with 10 days off for holidays. All of the concepts that she was to be taught were prescribed by the program director, with consistent implementation and other issues covered by her consultant. At no time were frontline therapists (also called tutors) allowed to make decisions regarding what concepts to teach. The therapists were carefully and constantly trained in exactly how to teach each of the individualized lessons for each skill or concept prescribed for Maggie. Many of the lessons were designed specifically for her, especially those that addressed eating problems. All of her lessons targeted the specific deficits she had displayed at the assessment. For example, if she was already able to label "cup," "shoe," and "apple," but not able to label "banana," "shirt," and "car," then her labeling lessons would target words such as "banana," "shirt," and "car." It was not simply a matter of teaching her random labels as they came up. A reward system was started to address the inappropriate behaviors, as well as systematic teaching of skills that could help her avoid those behaviors. Objectives were developed for each skill or concept that Maggie was to learn as she started her program. In all, 54 skill objectives were prescribed for her at the beginning of her program, and it was expected that Maggie would need a year to complete these objectives. New objectives were added throughout her program to advance her skills as she mastered existing objectives.

Maggie never attended a special education class of any kind during her time with Bridges or afterward.

January 2003 (3 Months of ABA)

Maggie had made excellent progress, especially in language. She had started to use words to ask for items consistently. She had increased her labeling of objects by 273%, from 15 to at least 41 object labels. She followed at least 18 directions (she had followed none during the assessment). She was now able to name people, colors, and shapes. She could answer when asked what her name was. Of her original 54 objectives, she had already completely met 12 and was ready to start 28 more, 9 months ahead of schedule. She still showed difficulty with lessons that addressed eating skills. Several of her eating skills lessons required desensitization procedures to build up a positive reinforcement history for tolerating food. Structured peer lessons teaching more complex social skills with a typically developing child were recommended for the next quarter. An additional 5 hours per week of therapy time was added to her program to allow structured peer play and the teaching of toileting skills. Inappropriate behaviors had already been reduced to very low levels.

March 2003 (6 Months of ABA)

Maggie continued to make excellent progress in all areas. Her food desensitization procedures were almost completed. She had started toilet training. She could now take off her pants and shirt when asked.

She had mastered compliance to directions for waiting, stopping, and coming when called. She could play independently without engaging in self-stimulatory behavior for at least 5 minutes and was working on doing this without an adult nearby. She responded to and initiated greetings when someone arrived or left. She stayed with adults when walking with them in the community, even when her hand was not held. She asked other people to wait when she was interrupted from a favored task appropriately. She also appropriately tolerated being denied the chance to tell others to wait for her. She imitated two-step gross motor movements when they were presented in a discrete manner and novel sequences of at least four-step movements when they were presented as a song or other typical toddler activity. She echoed novel phrases consisting of three single-syllable words. She took turns with other people and played at least two simple board games. She manded (asked) for a wide variety of items and receptively and expressively identified more than 100 items. She followed directions with "ing" words, both with pictures and in the natural environment. She followed novel three-step directions. She answered at least three common safety questions such as, "What is your name?" and "How old are you?" She demonstrated generalization of her labeling, requesting, and play skills, as well as many others. She had met more than half of all her original 54 objectives as well as half of the 28 objectives started in the prior quarter. She was ready to start 51 new objectives. She had turned 3 years old, and her program was now jointly funded by the Regional Center and her school district.

July 2003 (9 Months of ABA)

By this time, Maggie was frequently using spontaneous language to talk about items, shapes, colors, people, and possessions. She demonstrated language skills while she was playing as well as in structured activities. Maggie started working on community outings and more elaborate play for structured peer-play activities. She also started working on imitating facial expressions, reacting to facial expressions of other people, and reacting to novel incongruous activities and events. She improved her ability to tolerate being told "no" without protest. She was refining her play skills to include pretending with imaginary items. Some of her new language skills included identifying generalized objects as big and little and more and less than a given sample. She had mastered her first two pronouns and five prepositions.

She had mastered answering "yes–no" questions and was working on identifying objects by negation (Which one is not red?). Her spontaneous language now contained many sentences, as well as language that had not been specifically taught. She was starting to give novel answers to questions. This was particularly exciting because it showed that Maggie was learning in the natural environment. She was ready to start attending a regular education preschool with support provided by her Bridges ABA staff. At that time, her program hours were increased to 40 hours per week.

October 2003 (the 1-Year Mark)

Maggie made exceptional progress during her entire first year of ABA. She met 49 of her original 54 objectives (91%). Her language became much more frequent and complex. She used the toilet when taken. She had developed many social skills with her peers and had begun attending regular education preschool with support from people in her home program twice a week for a total of 5½ hours per week.

Years later, Maggie's mother made these comments about the halfway point:

> I found the best thing about ABA to be the growth Maggie made with us. It also gave us the behavioral tools to use with her brothers. Every week improvements could be seen, and the consistent and constant level of expectations were beneficial. I loved that parent input was valued and incorporated into the program when possible. The most difficult part was being chained to the house—an adult must be in the house during therapy time and that makes it very difficult to leave the house. Also simply having people in the home for 25–40 hours per week can be difficult.
>
> But the results were worth it—I feel you [Bridges] gave my daughter back to us. About halfway through the program we began to hope that she would "make it"—she would be one of the children that achieved a level of functioning that allowed her to live normally and independently and eventually lose her label.

January 2004 (15 Months of ABA)

By this time Maggie was attending regular education preschool twice each week for a total of 7 hours per week. Maggie had mastered many skills at school with an adult nearby. Among these were the ability to follow directions given to the group, to maintain conversations with peers for at least two exchanges, to raise her hand, to imitate her peers, and to initiate and remain engaged in parallel play. She also played interactively with peers and played appropriately with the toys in the classroom and on the playground. She independently transitioned in the classroom, attended to the teacher, waited in line, used the school restroom, and washed her hands. She sought attention appropriately from peers and teachers at school when she wanted something or needed help or a playmate. She demonstrated generalization of the language skills she had learned at home in the school environment, including her numbers, letters, colors, and shapes.

Recommendations for the following quarter addressed Maggie's ability to continue to do well in school even when the school support adult was farther away from her. Maggie continued to work on social skills with peers in the home environment as well as at school. Maggie showed greater skills with peers in the school environment than at home. Structured peer-play sessions were continued in the home environment as well as at school to ensure that Maggie acquired skills in both environments.

Language had continued to grow tremendously. Maggie could now describe pictures in detail, answer and ask various "wh" questions with discrimination, identify items by feature and function, answer conversational statements, and use adjectives. She continued to use more complete sentences in all speech. She continued to work on identifying the possessions and likely desires of other people and answering questions such as "What's wrong?" and "What's funny?" about novel events. She started to demonstrate observational learning skills—learning from watching other children learn.

April 2004 (18 Months of ABA)

At this time, Maggie was using many skills she had learned in a one-on-one format in other areas—in the structured peer-play setting, in the community, and at school. She was answering questions and statements from adults and peers. She conversed with adults and children both in the home and at school. She played appropriately (even with no support adult in sight) for long periods of time without engaging in self-stimulatory behaviors. She played interactively with a large variety of toys and in various activities with peers in all environments. She ate new, unfamiliar foods without protest and used utensils appropriately.

She initiated appropriate play even when she was unaware that she was being watched, rather than engaging in self-stimulatory behavior. In fact, self-stimulatory behaviors were not noted at all during the 3-month period since her last report. She had successfully completed her desensitization procedures for eating skills. She now ate a variety of foods. She allowed people to wash, brush, and cut her hair without protest. She brushed her teeth. She used all of these skills with her family and teachers as well as with her ABA staff. Toilet training had long since been completed, including for nighttime. Maggie started to learn more and more skills in the natural environment. She was making the transition from structured learning to learning as typical children do, by watching others. It was recommended that her regular education preschool time increase to 5 days a week (4 hours each day) with Bridges support. The balance of her day was spent working on social skills with peers and in the community and on eliminating the remaining functional and play skill deficits.

July 2004 (21 Months of ABA)

By this point Maggie had met 100% of all of her objectives that were 1 year old or older. Her rate of acquisition for new skills continued to accelerate because she had mastered 94% of the objectives started in the prior quarter 9 months ahead of schedule. Maggie used her new skills in the community and during structured peer-play sessions even if the therapist faded out of sight. Maggie was succeeding for most of her day at school without any support of adults in sight. Inappropriate behaviors in all environments had been comparable to those of typical peers for many months at this point.

October 2004 (2 Years of ABA—End of Program)

At the 2-year mark, Maggie was ready for us to fade out her program. She had met all of her objectives that were due at that time, as well as all objectives that had been started and that were not due yet. She showed strong generalization of skills with her family, during structured peer play, in the community, and at school, as well as the ability to learn in a natural environment with no artificial supports.

The team left the house for the last time. Tears were in everyone's eyes (even Maggie's) because all of us had been part of such an emotional journey with the best possible ending. Maggie acquired a new baby brother shortly after she finished with us. She was at the birth and found the entire thing fascinating. She says she loves her baby brother, her family, school, her friends, and her teacher. Maggie completed her preschool year and was enrolled in a regular education kindergarten in the fall of 2005 with no special education supports.

January 2007

I was able to see Maggie and her family in January 2007 to follow up on her progress. Maggie's mom shared a video of Maggie riding her horse and told me about the very normal life that Maggie enjoys today.

> When asked if there was a special moment that helped to define where Maggie is today, her mother said, "Last night she had a school play. She stood in front of a thousand strangers and did her part. She never missed a beat!"
>
> To a parent with a newly diagnosed child Maggie's mother offers this advice:
>
> "Do it! Stick with it and do not get frustrated. Get all the help you can. It is a great ride when you see all the improvement, and all the hopes that went away when you got the diagnosis start coming back, little by little, and when the door closes and the tutors go away, everyone looks at her and knows she did it for all the little things she learns every day."

Maggie continued to grow and learn after her program ended. She does not need any special education services, and there is no expectation that she will ever need them again. Her current teacher and principal are not aware of her earlier history.

While I was at the house, Maggie called from the school to say she had forgotten her lunch, so we went to the school to meet her and to give her lunch box to her. She did not remember me but was cheerful and polite. Her mother told Maggie that I was one of the people who had helped her when she was young. She smiled. I asked her if she was happy. Maggie simply looked surprised and said, "I'm very happy!"

So was I.

5

Hey, Look, It's a Train!

REBECCA P. F. MACDONALD

Jamie was a 3-year-old little boy who had recently been diagnosed with autism spectrum disorder when he first came to our school for an intake evaluation. He was one of triplets. His siblings were developing normally, but Jamie's language and social behavior were already quite delayed. Jamie was very interested in things that happened in his environment. During one of our initial assessments of Jamie, a therapist presented a tambourine to him, and he happily engaged with the toy by banging and shaking it. He looked at the toy and appeared to be enjoying the sensory experience of the noise and the tactile experience of banging. He, however, never looked up at the therapist to share the toy, nor did he hold up the toy to show it to the therapist. He was engaged in a solitary sensory experience, completely content to be in his own world. The therapist attempted to play with Jamie. He tolerated this intrusion but did not look up at the therapist until she removed the toy from him and waited for eye contact. He whined at the removal of the toy and eventually looked up at the therapist, who immediately re-presented the toy. He went back into solitary play, manipulating the tambourine and rhythmically bobbing his head to the noise he created.

Four years later, Jamie is entering second grade at his local public school, where he is fully included in academic and social activities along with his peers. He can read at grade level and can solve math problems in his head! Let's follow Jamie on his journey from that little 3-year-old who did not share his world with others to the second grader who enjoys talking about sports and interacting with friends.

For Jamie and so many other children with autism, a keenly developed repertoire of social skills is critical to their prognosis and success in later life. We will highlight the sequence of social behaviors that we taught Jamie over the years and emphasize the importance of creating a rich social environment to support and nurture the development of these skills. Joint attention responding and joint attention initiating are key features of our social skills curriculum.

Early Years

When we first met Jamie, he was not interested in the activities of the people around him. His language was not well developed. He infrequently used words to communicate with others but was able to label many objects in his environment. Jamie was showing deficits in joint attention.

Joint attention is the ability to coordinate attention between people and objects or events in order to share an awareness of these objects or events. Here is an example: A butterfly flies through the window into a young child's playroom. The child looks up, squeals with delight, points to the butterfly, and then shifts her gaze to Mom, who is also in the room. The mother looks from the child to the butterfly and says, "Yes, that's a butterfly, isn't she beautiful." The child looks back at the butterfly and smiles. This very natural event is a well-developed part of any typical child's social repertoire. A child's use of gaze shifts and gestures to share an interesting event is referred to as joint attention. Children with autism often show deficits in joint attention. The presence of an unexpected event in a child's environment, such as the appearance of the butterfly, may result in the child looking at the butterfly, but rarely will it result in sharing the experience with a caregiver. Appendix A provides additional information on joint attention and how to develop it.

Responding to Joint Attention

One of the earliest behaviors we targeted for Jamie was eye contact with familiar people in his environment. We first taught Jamie to look at us whenever we called his name. We sat knee to knee and reinforced him with a favorite treat every time he gave us eye contact in response to his name. We began with requiring only a fleeting glance and then over time required him to look at the therapist for up to 2 seconds. If at any point he did not look up, we would prompt him by tracking the treat from his face to ours. We paired the treat with lots of social praise and tickles in an effort to build a social rapport between Jamie and the therapist. When he was reliably looking at us in response to his name, we increased the difficulty of the task by giving Jamie a toy to play with and then intermittently calling his name. As before, we would reinforce him each time he looked at us in response to his name. As time went on, we no longer delivered treats, only social praise or tickles, and his performance maintained. We then gave Jamie a toy to play with and moved away from him. Though he could still see us, we were not directly in his field of vision. We again called his name and required him to look at us in response to his name, but now from a greater distance while he was occupied with a toy. We continued to increase the difficulty of the task by varying the settings and the therapist and then taught his parents how to get Jamie to look at them at home every time they called his name. This was now a well-established behavior in Jamie's social repertoire.

Sharing attention with another person requires not only establishing eye contact with that person but also being able to follow a person's point and gaze shift to something in the environment. This is called responding to joint attention. In this case, the familiar adult establishes eye contact with the child and then points and shifts the child's gaze to a toy in the environment. The goal is for the child to follow the adult's eye gaze to anywhere in the room. This might include the ceiling, the floor, or a shelf. To qualify as a well-established behavior, the child should engage in this behavior in the absence of an adult-delivered reinforcer, such as a treat or social praise.

Look What I See

After about 6 months of early intervention treatment, Jamie was now ready to learn joint attention skills. We began by teaching him not only to look at us but to follow our eye gaze paired with a point to a picture in a book. Initially we also paired the point with the word "look." Every time Jamie followed our gaze shift and pointed to a picture, we commented on the picture and reinforced him with a treat. This behavior quickly emerged in Jamie's repertoire. An added benefit of this procedure was that Jamie began to comment on the pictures in the book on his own. He initially repeated what the therapist said but over time made comments that were different from the therapist's.

We also used a more traditional discrete trial procedure to teach Jamie to follow an adult's gaze shift to a picture or object in his environment. For example, we sat at a small table across from Jamie. We arranged objects in various places within a 180-degree radius of him (e.g., to the left, right, and in front). As with the other procedures, we established eye contact with Jamie and said, "What am I looking at?" as we shifted our eyes (not our head) toward the toy or picture. If he was able to follow our gaze, he then said the name of the toy. We typically provided social praise and tokens or other identified reinforcers to reinforce this skill. As Jamie showed the ability to follow our eye gaze shifts, we moved away from the table to different locations around the room and then to different rooms. Eventually we made this a game and took turns with Jamie, having him say where we were looking and then having us say where he was looking. This proved to be an important part of establishing the social interaction and the social rapport necessary for more complex joint attention.

We postulate that following an adult's gaze shift or point is in fact compliance to the adult's directive for the child to look at something in the environment. The adult's gaze shift or point acquires control over the child's gaze shift response. The consequences that follow the child's gaze shift (i.e., the presence of a novel stimulus) reinforce the behavior. Teaching children to respond to more subtle joint attention bids, such as shifts in eye gaze, is important for increasing their social awareness.

The bigger challenge was to teach Jamie to follow our eye gaze to toys and pictures around the room without using a point or the word "look." Typical children learn quickly that much of the time it is worth their while to follow a caregiver's gaze because often that gaze indicates that something interesting is happening in their environment. For example, a mother might look in the direction of a puppy that is entering a room, an unexpected but interesting event. With enough exposure to these types of experiences, the child learns to follow the gaze shift of a caregiver much of the time. Our data from typical children indicate that even when the events that adults are looking at are not very interesting, typical children follow an adult's gaze more than 90% of the time.

Follow My Gaze: The Train Is Whistling!

One strategy we used with Jamie was based on just this notion that typical children learn to follow an adult gaze because it leads to something unexpected or interesting. We have found that by using toys that make noise we can teach the child to follow the eye gaze of an adult. Additionally, this response generalizes to untrained toys and settings. An artifact of this training has been an increase in the child's gaze shifts back to the adult as the interesting event is occurring.

We placed toys around the room that could be activated with a remote button, like a dog that barked and jumped or a train that lit up and whistled loudly. Jamie really enjoyed these kinds of toys regardless of how noisy or active they were. We set up these toys in four places around the room, in front, behind, and next to Jamie. Then we called his name. As soon as he looked at us, we shifted our gaze and head toward one of the toys. Whether he looked or not, we activated the toy, which always resulted in his looking at the toy. Jamie smiled and squealed with delight as the toys came alive. Over trials, we began to delay the time between our looking in the direction of the toy and our activating the toy. Eventually, Jamie was looking at the toy before we were scheduled to activate it. At this point, we activated the toy only contingent upon Jamie's following our gaze toward the toy. His face beamed! He was now looking back and forth between us and the toys on his own. He was truly enjoying this interaction with us.

After a year of early intensive intervention, the challenge that remained was to see if he would continue to follow our gaze shift to a variety of different toys even when they did not make noise or have moving parts. Jamie continued to follow our gaze as long as we occasionally included a toy that activated. We also wanted to know if Jamie could do this in the context of play. Again, our data from typical children indicate that even when they are playing with a toy, if an adult calls their name and shifts gaze toward something in the environment, they will look in the direction of the adult gaze more than 90% of the time, a very reliable behavior. We gave Jamie the opportunity to select a toy to play with and placed toys around the room. Although he did not follow our gaze shift every time we asked him to, he looked in the direction of our gaze shift much of the time. Jamie had learned to follow a caregiver's eye gaze to gain information about his environment. This skill is critical to the development of a more complex social repertoire.

Responding to Joint Attention During Conversations

Our next goal for Jamie was to be able to embed this new skill of following the eye gaze of an adult, in the context of a simple verbal exchange. Jamie had the language to be able to comment about things in his environment. He was learning to incorporate attributes, preposi-tions, and pronouns into his conversations with adults. During conver-sations, we required Jamie to look at the person he was talking to while that person was speaking to him and then while he was speak-ing. Once he learned this, we added the requirement that Jamie follow the adult's gaze shift to something in the environment. He was prompted to comment on the object the therapist was looking at in order for the conversation to continue. This skill took several months to acquire, but, once he had mastered it, he enjoyed the social exchange. He was now responding to the joint attention bids of adults in many different situations and was doing this in the context of natu-rally occurring consequences.

Joint Attention Initiations

One day, during Jamie's second year at our school, I was watching him in the integrated preschool classroom, where he was sitting at a table between two typical peers. They were involved in an art activity, and Jamie was sitting quietly, looking at the work in front of him. Although this seemed like very appropriate behavior, it struck me that Jamie never looked up at his peers or his teacher. His focus was solely on the project at hand. As I surveyed the classroom, the other children were all busy chatting with each other and looking between their projects and their therapist and peers. They were initiating joint attention by showing their peers their work and commenting about the colors they were using and making their needs known to their therapist by looking at them and clearly requesting things. Jamie was doing none of these things. He remained in his own world. We still had much work to do to help Jamie connect with the people around him.

The behaviors we had taught Jamie so far fall into the category of joint attention responding. This means that he will respond to an adult's bid for him to look at something that the adult is looking at. This is different from joint attention initiation, in which the child initi-ates a bid for the adult to look at something the child is interested in. For example, a child sees a helicopter flying loud and low in the sky and uses a gesture to point out the helicopter. The child then verifies that the adult has seen the helicopter by looking at the helicopter and then the adult and back to the helicopter. Using a behavioral frame-work, we might say that at the onset of the interesting event, in this case the helicopter, the child has a choice regarding behavior allocation. He can engage solely in the behavior that produces event-related consequences (watching and enjoying the loud helicopter), or he can engage in both event-related behavior and joint attention initiation (sharing the event by looking back at the adult, pointing, and commenting on the helicopter) in order to obtain both event-related reinforcement and social reinforcement. We refer to the latter as shared attention or the initiating of joint attention.

Initiating joint attention involves getting another person's attention. One of the characteristics of children with autism is that they tend to gain access to things by taking an adult's hand and leading the adult to what they want. Coordinated eye contact and language are typically not a part of these interactions. It is important that children with autism be taught to gain an adult's attention first when requesting something from another person. This is a prerequisite to initiating joint attention to share something of interest.

During Jamie's second year of intervention, we taught him to request preferred items using a coordinated eye gaze in combination with a point gesture. Jamie rarely looked at an adult when he was requesting something. He would often begin by looking at the object he wanted. He might then label the object and reach for it. Indeed, he was quite persistent at making these types of requests in the absence of any eye contact. Our first job was to teach Jamie how to make simple requests using coordinated eye contact. We accomplished this by presenting a toy he preferred and making the establishment of eye contact with us a requirement for access to the toy. We presented his favorite stuffed bear, which he reached for, but we kept it out of his field of grasp until he looked up at the teacher. It took many trials for him to learn that he had to look at us every time he requested something. Eventually, this became a part of his requesting repertoire, and we moved on to using coordinated eye contact in the presence of choice making.

Which One Do You Want?

Life is full of opportunities for us to make simple choices. Embedding a request with coordinated eye contact into this choice making allows for a social interaction. To teach this, we showed Jamie two of his preferred treats and had him look at the one he wanted. We began by allowing him access to the one he looked at, and then we added the requirement that he look at the item and shift his gaze to look at his therapist to request the item. We prompted by tracking, which involved using the item he was looking at and moving it from his gaze direction to our eyes. As soon as he looked at the therapist, he received the item. Once this was established, we introduced a gesture and then the words "I want that one." Jamie was now required to look at the item he wanted, look back at the therapist, then point to the item he chose and say "I want that one." Gaze shifting back and forth between the requested item and the adult was a critical aspect of this social response. We wanted Jamie to use his eyes and gestures to initiate the request, rather than labeling the item, because more advanced joint attention requires these two skills.

Soliciting Attention to Request

Often, when a child wants to either request something or share something he sees with another person, he does not persist in trying to get the attention of that person. There are a variety of ways to teach children to persist. We began by teaching Jamie to tap the person's shoulder to get her attention and to wait until the person looked at him to initiate the request. One of the simplest ways to start to teach this behavior was to stage situations in which Jamie needed to make a request from an adult to access more of something he wanted. Snack time proved to be a perfect scenario. Jamie was seated at the snack table, with a few pieces of popcorn on his plate. The therapist was seated next to him. Jamie generally would just call out what he wanted or grab things. If he did either to indicate he wanted more, the therapist prompted him to tap her shoulder to gain her attention. She then looked at him and verbally modeled, "Popcorn, please." When he established eye contact with the therapist and made the verbal request, she gave him more popcorn. He quickly learned this skill in the context of snack time.

Gaining a person's attention in order to make a request involves discriminating whether the person can be interrupted and then making the initiation. It is often necessary to formally teach this discrimination. We selected a variety of situations to teach this discrimination to Jamie. The first situation involved having the therapist positioned so that her back was toward Jamie. He was required to tap her shoulder and wait for her to turn around and give eye contact. Another situation required the adult to be busy on a task, which meant that Jamie had a choice: wait until the adult was done with the task or interrupt the adult by tapping on her shoulder. In the latter case, when the adult said she was busy, Jamie was required to wait until she was ready. A third scenario involved having the adult talking with another adult. As with many new behaviors for children with autism, this skill did not generalize to new people in novel situations. We needed to teach Jamie how and when to gain the attention of others; it required the use of multiple people across many situations and settings before the behavior occurred in new and novel situations.

Looking at and Pointing to Pictures in a Book

By the end of Jamie's second year of intervention, we focused on expanding his joint attention initiation skills. Jamie really enjoyed books, so we began teaching him to initiate to us through the use of books. Children's books are full of colorful pictures to talk about and therefore are a wonderful medium to use for beginning to teach joint attention initiating. Initiating joint attention involves a complex set of behaviors, including pointing, eye gaze shifting, and commenting.

Using a photo album, we made a book specifically for Jamie that had pictures of things he enjoyed, such as animals and trains. We put one picture on each page. It was large and colorful. We began a teaching session by opening up the book and guiding Jamie's finger to point to the picture while he looked at the picture. We commented on the picture ("What a big shiny red engine!") and reinforced him with tickles and social praise for pointing and looking. When he was able to do this each time we turned the page, we added the response of looking from the picture to us before we reinforced him. To help him learn this response, we used our hand to track his eyes from the picture to our eyes. He was now able to point to the picture and look back at the therapist reliably every time a new picture was shown to him. Our last task was to teach him to comment on the picture. With only a few verbal prompts and a wait of a few seconds, Jamie quickly learned to comment on the picture. As time went by, Jamie made many comments about the picture, using the language we had taught him. He could comment on the colors, size, and actions of the figures shown in the pictures. Perhaps the most important change in Jamie's interaction with the therapist was his overall affect. He was now smiling, commenting and using gaze shifts to interact with the therapist and to share the pictures in the book with someone. He seemed genuinely happy during these interactions. He was beginning to show joint attention in this very simple context. Though we knew we still had much work to do, we were very excited for Jamie.

Taking this complex set of behaviors from a book to other situations in Jamie's day was no simple matter. We began by moving from our simple photo albums to picture books in his classroom. In the context of reading in the book area or at a table in the middle of the classroom, we required the same set of responses. He learned quickly to point to pictures in lots of books, look back at his therapist, and comment on the picture. He could do this without explicit reinforcement, but these actions occurred in the context of the therapist's natural social interactions, including comments and smiles. Jamie also had a very keen sense of humor, and the interactions were often characterized by his teasing or fooling the therapist by saying something silly about the picture.

As in the butterfly example, typically developing children comment on naturally occurring unexpected events in their environment. To simulate this for Jamie, we extended the book picture task to pictures around his classroom. We placed a variety of pictures, some of Jamie and some of other children he knew, doing things throughout his classroom and in the hallway in his school. We brought Jamie around the classroom and stopped at the pictures and waited. If he did not initiate joint attention by pointing to the picture and commenting on it, we prompted this behavior. Because he already had learned these skills in a more structured teaching format, he quickly began to initiate joint attention with these pictures. Jamie was now initiating joint attention in the context of pictures both in a book and throughout his classroom environment, but he was still not initiating joint attention during play.

Interestingly, both joint attention and play emerge in the same developmental time frame, and both are linked to language. Pretend play is one of the hallmarks of childhood play, yet children with autism rarely engage in play that has these pretend qualities. One of the earliest strategies we used to teach Jamie these pretend play skills was to teach him how to do simple and complex actions with toys. For example, we taught him to feed a baby doll, to drive a car up a ramp, and to make a toy frog hop. We then added sound effects to each of these actions, for example, by making a car noise as the car drove up the ramp. We then added more actions to these events: for example, the car drove up the ramp, and then the man put gas in the car and then went to the car wash. Jamie enjoyed playing in this manner but continued to play in a very solitary way. The fact that he did enjoy playing, however, gave him the foundation to start to introduce joint attention into the context of play.

Show During Play

We have found that a mystery box is a wonderful toy to teach children with autism to show things in their environment to others. A mystery box is filled with lots of interesting objects, and the game involves taking turns with an adult. Jamie already knew how to take turns from his experience playing games in his classroom. The rules of the game were that Jamie had to pull an object out of the mystery box, hold it up in front of the therapist, and look from the toy to the therapist while making a comment about the toy. He could then play with the toy or give the therapist a turn. In the beginning, the therapist needed to prompt Jamie to hold the toy up in front of the therapist. She did this by tapping or holding his elbow and then his wrist until he was able to do this independently. We made sure the box was full of toys that Jamie could label and talk about. As he became more proficient at this game, we moved to a commercially available toy called Ned's Head. Ned's Head was full of all sorts of gross objects, like vomit, a cotton swab with ear wax on it, and large, ugly bugs. Jamie, with his sense of humor, loved this game! As Jamie entered his third year of treatment, he had developed nice pretend-play skills and a rich repertoire of language and was beginning to share his day with others by showing and talking about toys in his classroom.

Look What I Did!

We now wanted Jamie to solicit our attention to show us something he had built during play. He loved to build creatures using K'NEX plastic pieces. He could look at a picture of a sea creature and build it, using all the pieces. We then taught him to show us his creation by holding it up in front of us and saying, "Look what I made!" He required prompting initially, but, because he loved the attention he got from showing us what he had built, he quickly began using this strategy not only in the context of these creatures but in the context of lots of things he did during his day. He was now using joint attention to gain our attention and share his accomplishments with us.

At our school, there is a train that passes by quite close to the building each day. This train is visible from the window in the classroom, and children can not only see it but feel the rumbling and hear the whistle. One of the most exciting moments for us was the day Jamie noticed the train. He looked at and pointed to the train, then looked at his therapist and pointed to the train, yelling, "Hey, look, it's a train!" He was initiating joint attention on his own. He was sharing the excitement of the train with teachers and peers in his classroom.

Listening to a Conversation

As Jamie became more connected with people in his classroom and communicated more with people throughout his day, we began working on making sure he was listening during conversational exchanges. This is an important skill because, in order to participate in a social group, one must be able to listen to more than one conversational partner. We asked Jamie to listen to two people talk about what they had done on the weekend. At first, he did not look at the people when they were speaking. He also could not answer questions about what they had said. To help him focus on listening to the person who was talking, we had that person hold a ball in his hand and told Jamie to follow the ball. Some additional gestural prompts were required for him to look at the person who had the ball in his hand, but he learned this quickly. With the additional requirement that he look at the person who was speaking, he was attending and listening to the conversation. He could now answer questions about what the person had said. He could even now participate and add information about what he had done on the weekend.

By the end of Jamie's third year of EIBI, we began integrating him into his local kindergarten classroom. While there were many opportunities for Jamie to use his joint attention skills in the new classroom, he required prompting. In addition, we were finding that he was not using his joint attention skills in the context of social conversations with adults or peers. This remained an area for us to address specifically in the kindergarten classroom.

Joint Attention During a Conversation

Because the goal of joint attention is to be able to share information about a topic of interest to the speaker and another person, we first established topics of conversation that might be common between Jamie and his peers. Jamie was particularly interested in sports. He loved to talk about sports statistics, players, and teams. One way to structure this conversation was to use a sports magazine. Coordinated joint attention in the context of a magazine can involve many behaviors. We taught Jamie to point to pictures in the magazine to show us something he wanted to talk about. We also taught Jamie to hold up a page in the magazine to show us something of interest to him. He could talk about specific players and how they had done in a game over the weekend. We required him to look at us while he was talking and to coordinate showing or gesturing to the pictures during these exchanges. Because this was a topic of great interest to Jamie, he was very animated as he spoke. He was now sharing something of interest to him with others in his environment. Indeed, we had come a long way in 3 years.

What We Have Learned

The role of applied behavior analysts has always been one of addressing socially important behaviors. We know that a diagnosis of autism does not predict the outcome for an individual child or that child's potential responsiveness to treatment. Some children make dramatic gains, and some do not. So, what are those early behavioral indicators that might account for these differences in responsiveness to treatment? One early deficit that has surfaced as being critical to the prognosis for progress of children on the autism spectrum concerns the development of joint attention.

Perhaps even more important to the field of autism is the formulation of a model for the analysis of joint attention. Gaining a better understanding of the behavioral contingencies that are involved in the development and maintenance of joint attention initiation, we believe, will lead to more effective treatment. Because we are talking about social behavior, we are looking for changes not only in the target behaviors but in other, nontargeted social behaviors that make up the rich repertoire of spontaneous joint attention behaviors seen in young, typically developing infants and children. Through our systematic work with Jamie, he has acquired a repertoire of social skills that he now uses because he wants to share his world with others.

6

Good Golly Miss Molly!

AUDREY GIFFORD

At a local elementary school, wobbly lines of laughing, chattering, gap-toothed 6-year-olds sort themselves into clumps of boys and girls at the entrance to the cafeteria each day at lunch. Molly is shorter than the rest—tiny, blond, and dynamic. She is always surrounded by a crowd of other little girls, and they talk and giggle endlessly. She is very sociable and is wonderful with both old friends and new classmates.

Molly wants to be a first-grade teacher and a mom when she grows up. Even though she is barely old enough to be in first grade, she does very well. She is in the chess club (and beats the third graders!) and the science club at school. Her first-grade teacher says there are no issues in the classroom and told her mother she did not even need the usual parent-teacher conference.

At home Molly is happy and well adjusted. She plays alone as well as with friends and with her brother. She often sings to herself, as little girls do. She has a phenomenal memory for music and can repeat a song perfectly after hearing it only once. Molly also deals with the challenges of being a sibling to a child with autism. Often she plays very well and patiently with her brother, but she will let her parents know when she has had enough and needs a break. Like many siblings of children with autism, she sometimes finds herself taking on a nurturing role. She helps keep her brother busy and on task at home when he might otherwise fall into inappropriate behaviors. Her older brother is fully included (with support) in regular education classes at her school. Sometimes Molly is embarrassed by her brother at school, but she stands up for him to the other children. Last year, a much taller child in her class said to her, "I don't have to be partners with your brother!" Tiny kindergartener Molly put her hands on her hips, looked *way* up at the other girl, and scolded, "If you don't play with my brother, then I will not play with you!"

Molly is invited to a lot of birthday parties and enjoys all of the activities, including the Happy Birthday song. But at one time, tolerating that song was a challenge so severe that it took Molly almost 2 years to be able to hear it without screaming. Only a few of us know that Molly herself was diagnosed with autism when she was a very young child. Certainly none of the children she plays with (or their parents) know.

The Early Years

As a very young infant, Molly screamed very often. Some days, it was almost constant. At 18 months, she could not ask for items or name common objects such as shoes or cups. But, even at that age, Molly could name numbers and letters. After a routine 18-month checkup revealed some concerns, she was evaluated for autism by Dr. Linda Copland of Kaiser Permanente. In the waiting room for the evaluation, Molly was fascinated by a sippy cup held by another child. She showed no interest in the other child. Dr. Copland noted that at the evaluation Molly displayed fleeting eye contact, was shy, got upset when praised, resisted language tasks by covering her face or turning to her dad, could not follow directions, showed no thematic sequential play with toys, and showed no pointing to establish joint attention. The doctor also noted a lack of functional use of language, as well as the reciting of letters and numbers in a noncommunicative way. Molly was reported to be able to point to pictures when asked by her family. She did not do that when asked by the doctor. She did not tolerate having a story read to her. She could identify one body part (tummy) but not her nose. It was noted that she hid her eyes around new places and did not use words even when they were in her vocabulary. She was reported to have had about 22 words at that time. She did not point to any object on request, match, or follow directions. She perseverated on nesting cups for a considerable amount of time and became upset when they were removed. She whined and turned her head to her dad's chest when praised and applauded.

TESTING DATA FOR MOLLY*

Developmental Domain	Standard Score	Age Equivalent (Months)	Test Name
Mental age	73	15–16 months	BAYLEY
Communication	76	Not stated	VABS
Daily living skills	72	Not stated	VABS
Social	83	Not stated	VABS
Motor skills	103	Not stated	VABS
Adaptive behavior composite	78	Not stated	VABS

*Molly was 1 year, 6 months, and 22 days old at the time these tests were administered (June 19, 2002).
Bayley (Bayley Scales of Infant Development)
VABS (Vineland Adaptive Behavior Scales—Interview Edition, Expanded Form)

MOLLY'S PRESENTING SYMPTOMS THAT MET *DSM-IV* CRITERIA FOR AUTISTIC DISORDER

1. Failure to develop peer relationships appropriate to developmental level.
2. Delay in, or total lack of, the development of spoken language (not accompanied by an attempt to compensate through alternative modes of communication such as gesture or mime).
3. Lack of varied, spontaneous make-believe play or social imitative play appropriate to developmental level.
4. Encompassing preoccupation with one or more stereotyped and restricted patterns of interest that is abnormal either in intensity or in focus.

Dr. Copland administered three tests to Molly—the Bayley Scales of Infant Development, the Vineland Adaptive Behavior Scales (see the table above), and the Childhood Autism Rating Scale (CARS). She noted that Molly's Bayley score was brought down primarily by language deficits and deficits in thematic sequential play and imitation. It was noted that her scores on the Vineland seemed to underestimate her level of disability. Her CARS scores (31.5) placed her in the autistic spectrum disorder range. On the basis of a number of presenting symptoms (see the table below), Dr. Copland diagnosed Molly with PDD-NOS.[13] That diagnosis was refined 1 year later to autism by Dr. Phyllis Magnani at Alta California Regional Center.

---

13 Pervasive developmental disorder, not otherwise specified—one of the autistic spectrum disorders.

July 22, 2002 (20 Months Old)

A report was issued by Rose Godfrey, a speech-language pathologist, about an evaluation of Molly's language skills. She was 20 months old at the time of her evaluation. Molly was tested on the Bzoch-League Receptive-Expressive Emergent Language Test (REEL-2). This showed scores of receptive language of 12–14 months and expressive language of 14–16 months.

The Call to Us

We already were providing services to Molly's older brother, so the family knew about ABA (Applied Behavior Analysis). Molly's devastated father called us on the day Molly was diagnosed, and we were able to schedule an assessment for her within a few weeks. The family had originally been told about ABA by Suzanne Cooper, a service coordinator at Alta California Regional Center. Ms. Cooper was able to speed Molly through the intake process at Alta California Regional Center so that services could begin very quickly.

August 2002

Molly was 20 months old at the time of her assessment. She was tiny for her age. She touched things in a very tentative, delicate manner. Her touch was so delicate that it was speculated that some of her receptive language skills were masked because Molly simply did not like the sensation of touching things, even pictures. Receptive language (what someone understands) is often measured by having the person touch or point to the picture someone is naming. For a long time, Molly had a strong aversion to tactile sensation on her hands, and this led us to create modifications such as padding the handles on her scissors as she progressed through her therapy. She vigorously protested holding hands, as well as any prompts (help) that involved touching her hands.

At the time she was assessed, Molly was unable to communicate her wants and needs, even though she was able to count objects. In fact, naming numbers and letters was observed to be a self-stimulatory behavior, because she recited them over and over. This sort of perseverative behavior is very common in children with autism. She was prescribed a PECS (picture exchange communication system) book to give her a way to communicate her desires. This let her hand a picture of the desired item to an adult so that she could ask for something without talking and it was used as a bridge to having her ask for items with spoken words.

Molly spent much of the assessment time resisting our attempts to get her to do things. Sometimes she simply did not respond. Other times she shouted no, screamed, ran away, deliberately fell down, and cried. She said "owie" repeatedly and ran to her parents when a person entered the house, as well as when she was frustrated or seemed to want attention. Molly spoke during the assessment, usually to say the names of items. She became upset if she was not acknowledged after she named an item. She named more numbers and letters (42) than common objects (36). She did not use her language to talk to people or to ask for items. Molly had a harder time receptively identifying objects than she did naming objects. Molly matched items and pictures very well. Molly named seven shapes but no colors. She used no verbs at any time. Molly stacked blocks very well, but this activity became perseverative, and it was difficult to distract her from it. She looked at books, rolled cars, pushed buttons on toys, and played with a Mr. Potato Head. She completed single inset puzzles if motivated—a big wooden shape puzzle was a favorite.

After reviewing the data from her initial assessment, we prescribed 20 hours per week of ABA for Molly. We opted for this low number of hours because Molly took two naps per day and was still very young. Additionally, she was prescribed 5 hours per month of direct supervision by a program director with a master's degree and several years' experience and 15 hours per month of supervision by a consultant with a bachelor's degree as well as several years' experience. Her program was implemented 52 weeks a year with 10 days off for holidays. All of the concepts that she was to be taught were prescribed by the program director. Consistent implementation and other issues were covered by her consultant. At no time were frontline therapists (also called tutors) allowed to make decisions regarding what concepts to teach. The therapists were carefully and constantly trained in exactly how to teach each of the individualized lessons prescribed for Molly. Objectives were developed for each skill or concept that Molly was to learn as she started her program. In all, 40 skill objectives (such as labeling colors and verbs, asking for items or activities, dressing, and following directions) were prescribed for her at the beginning of her program. We expected that Molly would need a year to complete these objectives. New objectives were added throughout her program to advance her skills as she mastered older objectives.

Molly never attended a special education class of any kind during her time with Bridges or afterward. Below is a reflection of Molly's experience at the in-house program provided by Bridges.

> Molly's program started in September of 2002. When Molly was asked what she remembers about the program she mentioned painting toenails (an activity used as a reinforcer for her at the end of her program). Ironically, Molly needed a desensitization program at the beginning of her ABA therapy to allow anyone to trim her toenails, yet she eventually found that sort of activity so much fun she would work to be able to do it!
>
> When Molly's mother was asked about the beginning of the program, she remembered Molly screaming. There was lots and lots of screaming. It took several weeks of therapy for Molly to learn to tolerate being asked to do things, but by the end of the first month she was doing quite well and was usually compliant, especially given her age.

November 2002 (2 Months of ABA)

After 2 months, an update report was prepared. Molly had made extremely good progress. She was demonstrating much better receptive (and expressive) language skills, and perseveration on letters and numbers was much reduced. She continued to have issues around tactile defensiveness, especially in her hands. Molly was now typically using one- to two-word sentences in spontaneous speech and had initiated social play at least once. Molly had already met 14 of her original 40 objectives, 10 months ahead of schedule. She started 33 more in the next 3 months. A structured peer-play component was also incorporated into her program at this time.

A disastrous trip to buy a family Christmas tree had resulted in Molly's screaming in terror when she saw the flashing lights. After that, she screamed instantly if she saw flashing lights. In order to address this, we added a systematic desensitization program to her therapy. This involved exposing Molly to flashing lights for very short time periods (such as 5 seconds) while heavily reinforcing her when she did not scream. This procedure was done once each day. Every time that Molly met the criteria for mastery at a given time interval, the amount of time she needed to tolerate the lights was increased slightly.

March 2003 (6 Months of ABA)

At the 6-month point, Molly had met 27 of her original 40 goals, 5 months ahead of schedule. She demonstrated vastly improved language skills. Her basic language was again tested formally by another speech-language pathologist, Mary Currier, MS, CCC-SLP (see the table below). Molly tested at or above chronological age levels in most language areas. She scored at the 3-year-old level in understanding single words, even though she was only 27 months old. Her receptive language skills tested at the 37-month age level. This was at the high end of normal and showed 21 months of growth during the 6 months she had been in the program. Her expressive language scored at the 29-month level. This was also in the normal range and showed that Molly had made 15 months of growth during the 6 months she had been in the program. Functional use of language was still a problem for Molly. She still had difficulty following directions, turning when her name was called, referring to herself as "I" or "me" rather than in the third person, and using "mine." She did not use sentences to make requests or comments. Instead, she used small chunks of information to request an activity. For example, when requesting to bounce on a ball she said, "Mulberry Bush," which was the song usually played for her while she was bouncing on the ball.

MOLLY'S TESTING DATA AFTER 6 MONTHS OF ABA

Molly's test results from examination on March 3, 2003 (age 27 months):

Peabody Picture Vocabulary Test—revised (PPVT-R), form L

This showed a raw score of 24 and a standard score of 111. This placed Molly in the 77th percentile, with an age equivalent of 3 years.

Preschool Language Scale-3 (PLS-3) Auditory comprehension

This showed a raw score of 31 and a standard score of 115. This indicated an age equivalent of 37 months.
Notes: Molly excelled at colors, verbs, parts of a whole, and attributes. However, other skills more typical of children her age posed greater difficulty, including understanding of groups of objects, negation, and making inferences.

Preschool Language Scale-3 (PLS-3) Expressive language

This showed a raw score of 22 and a standard score of 890. This indicated an age equivalent of 29 months.

Note. Molly could not speak about her mom, dad, or brother with more than one to two prompts without visual cueing also no possessives. Articulation was noted as appropriate.

One of the challenges Molly faced was tolerating people singing. In particular, Molly screamed and cried immediately whenever anyone tried to sing the Happy Birthday song. This was so pronounced that at her own birthday party the song was skipped entirely, and at other birthday celebrations Molly needed to be taken out of the room to avoid disrupting the party. We started a program to desensitize her to people singing (and to the Happy Birthday song in particular). At the beginning, Molly could tolerate only 1 second of the Happy Birthday song without screaming.

In March, an illness left Molly unable to participate in therapy for a week. She was very resistant to the demands of her program when she restarted. We had noticed that Molly was quite compliant when she did not seem to perceive a situation as a "demand" situation. When she *did* perceive something as a demand, she simply did not answer and resisted all prompts. She was still very young—not yet 2½. Because of her age, her program was already less formally structured than that typically used with an older child (such as her brother). She was always taught using behaviorally sound methodology, but the lessons were presented to her primarily while she and the therapist were sitting on the floor, engaged in games and other play-type activities. At this point, however, these modifications did not seem to be effective, so we changed the format of her program. We used unstructured time as a reward for responding to structured tasks. For example, when Molly answered one question in a structured format, she was allowed to spend the next 15–30 minutes in an unstructured format. During unstructured time, she was allowed to "take the lead" on the activity, while we "snuck in" the targeted lessons as they were appropriate to the activity. After the allotted time was over, she was again asked to answer one "structured" question. Each day, as she demonstrated success with structured questions, we gradually added a higher component of demand to her day. While these procedures were effective, it took several months for Molly to tolerate demand at her previous levels.

September 2003—The 1-Year Mark

By the 1-year mark, Molly had met all but two (95%) of her original objectives. She was still 2 months shy of her third birthday. Molly responded well to therapy at this point and tolerated high demand levels with few compliance problems. Her therapy concentrated on generalizing her skills to new environments and improving her ability to behave appropriately in the community, especially in new places. Pragmatic areas of language were still a concern, including initiation of speech, maintaining a conversation, and speaking to peers. We introduced new lessons to increase her use of language in a variety of environments and circumstances. Some of these addressed participating in true conversations, answering statements (not just questions), and using more skills with typically developing peers.

November 2003 (14 Months of ABA)

As Molly neared her third birthday the compliance issues returned with a vengeance. The old problem behaviors reappeared, but under different circumstances. We had first observed these behaviors when Molly was asked to do something—being "under demand." They had responded well to the procedures used in the spring. Now the behaviors did not occur when Molly was under demand; they occurred when the environment changed. Molly screamed, cried, fell down, ran away, and simply did not respond at all to anyone when something in the environment changed. The environmental changes that caused these behaviors were very minor, such as a dropped toy, a grandparent leaving the house, a popsicle being the "wrong" color, or other small events along those lines. It was observed that sometimes when these behaviors happened, it was possible to return the environment to the way it had been before. For example, if a toy fell and Molly started to scream, an adult sometimes put the toy back on the shelf. This made Molly stop screaming (which the adult wanted) and got the toy back on the shelf (which Molly wanted). It was, however, a recipe for a huge increase in these behaviors. Even when the environment was not changed back to its original condition, Molly sometimes closed her eyes or looked away from the item while she kept screaming.

These problem behaviors came at a particularly bad time. Molly had excellent language skills and was ready to start adding some time at a typical preschool to her program, with support provided by her in-home ABA staff. She also was ready to start working on toileting skills, and these behaviors did not bode well for a successful toilet-training experience or school.

A formal behavior plan was prepared for Molly. This included a detailed analysis of what happened before and after inappropriate behaviors occurred and allowed us to prescribe several strategies to treat the behaviors. All of the behaviors observed occurred when the environment changed. Interestingly, none occurred when Molly was "under demand." We hypothesized that Molly was using the behaviors to try to get the environment changed back to the way it had been before. To address this problem, we taught Molly a number of new skills. We also strengthened her existing skill of asking adults to move items appropriately. Some of the new skills she learned included asking adults to wait before they changed the environment, telling adults what to do under certain circumstances, and telling people she was mad. She was also given the chance to choose which lesson to work on (though she could not avoid any lesson altogether).

December 2003 (the Halfway Point)

Molly's mother remembers worrying that the funding agencies would decide Molly was not progressing well because of the tantrum behaviors, and that she might lose her services. She had a very difficult time with two children in the autism spectrum. The organizational and other responsibilities of having two full-time therapy programs in her house simultaneously were a huge strain.

But she also remembers all the help the therapy gave her in raising her children. The therapists became almost like part of the family. She learned strategies that helped immensely with both children. The programs taught everyone. Not long after this point in the program, Molly started to make great strides again. Every day she came closer to what her mother had dreamed she would be when she was a baby, before she was diagnosed.

By the end of December, the new plan had been in place for a month, and the inappropriate behaviors had disappeared completely. Even the trip to the Christmas tree lot was a pleasant holiday experience for the whole family.

February 2004 (17 Months in the Program)

Molly's inappropriate behaviors had decreased dramatically in all environments. None had occurred for 2 months. Molly continued to increase her ability to tolerate the normal environmental events that she previously seemed to find aversive. In February, she started a supported part-time regular education preschool placement two mornings a week with support from her Bridges staff. School and community skills, social skills with peers, and toileting were the primary focus of her program at this point.

Molly could now maintain appropriate conversations with adults and peers without help. She behaved appropriately in all community environments and had made very good progress on her social skills with peers. Despite her high skill levels in these areas, toileting remained very challenging. It was speculated that Molly was once again asserting her control over the situation. After all, Molly was the only one who could make herself urinate, and Molly undoubtedly knew that. We tried taking her to the bathroom on a regular schedule. She simply waited until all the therapists left and then had an accident. We then tried taking her to the bathroom only when she asked to go, to eliminate any control issues. Again, Molly simply waited until everyone left and then had an accident. Finally we decided to have a "potty week." During the "potty week," Molly stayed home from school, and the entire week was spent in or close to the bathroom. She was taken to the bathroom very frequently, with trips to the toilet every 30 minutes during the day. Between trips to the bathroom, she stayed close to the bathroom door. She wore only a shirt and her underwear, in order to quickly catch any potty opportunities between scheduled trips to the bathroom. Molly managed to not urinate at all (including at night) for more than 45 hours. At that point (when the adult who was with her had to leave for a moment to go to the bathroom), she "let loose" and had an accident. She waited more than 24 hours before urinating again. It seemed likely that the potty week would be a failure. Then, the next day, Molly urinated in the toilet, and by the end of the week she consistently stayed dry as long as we reminded her to use the bathroom regularly.

June 2004 (21 Months in the Program)

Molly had blossomed. She did so well in her part-time supported preschool placement that she increased her time at school from 2 to 4 days per week. The bulk of her Bridges program now took place at school. School was where the remaining issues of peer interaction and social skills were best taught. Molly put her hand over her face when given undesired instructions a few times at the beginning of the school year. These behaviors were ignored, and she was reinforced when she did respond appropriately to less-preferred instructions. The behavior completely disappeared after several weeks. She continued to show age-appropriate (or better) levels of unacceptable behaviors. She tolerated the Happy Birthday song all the way through without protest at school both times it was sung.

July 2004 (22 Months in the Program)

Molly was making excellent progress in all areas. She was now completely independent in her toileting skills, including at night. Casual observers would be very unlikely to see Molly as disabled most of the time at school, in the home, or in the community. In July, a new and frightening behavior emerged. Molly started to bite her own hand. She also started to call out in circle time at school to a degree that was disrupting the class. An emergency plan was put into place for the hand biting. The amount of reinforcement for refraining from biting was increased. We also prompted and reinforced a higher level of appropriate attention-seeking behavior. The descriptions of the behaviors suggested that a wish for adult attention was probably behind the biting and calling-out behaviors. If Molly used appropriate methods to get adult attention, she would have less reason to use hand biting and calling out to get this attention. Within days, the behavior disappeared. Again, Molly had let us know just who she felt should be in charge.

August 2004 (23 Months in the Program)

In August, other serious behavioral issues emerged. Molly had learned that if she screamed in the car, her brother would start to hit his head on the car window. Molly's brother had hit the window so hard that the family was seriously concerned that he could hurt himself—at one point they thought he could break the window with the force of the blow. Simple reward systems for increasingly difficult targets were prepared and given to Molly's grandmother and her mother. This was effective, and the behavior disappeared.

Molly had done so very well overall that it was easy to forget that she was still only 3 years old. She had not only her own issues to overcome but also the challenges of being a sibling to another young child with autism. As the new school year started, Molly continued to do very well at school. She was moved up to the older (3½ and 4-year-olds) pre-school classroom. After the initial start in the new class, she showed complete independence there, both during the academic instruction and in social interactions with peers and teachers. Because of her independence, the therapists' prompting was faded completely, and their role was shifted to monitoring her skills in the classroom and playground when Molly was not aware of their presence. This was done to make sure that the skills Molly exhibited with the therapists were maintained even when she was not aware that a therapist was present. The therapy she received after school between August and January was devoted almost entirely to improving her social skills.

Molly now consistently tolerated without protest the Happy Birthday song when it was sung for other children.

January 2005 (28 Months in the Program)

Molly completed the transition to independence at school. Molly attended preschool five mornings a week at a local private preschool for typically developing children. Molly no longer displayed inappropriate behaviors beyond those expected for a typical child her age at school, with peers, or in the community. Support staff no longer attended school with her. Continued observations by supervision staff and reports from her teacher and parents agreed that Molly was not distinguishable from her peers in the school and peer environments.

By mid-January, Molly had completed the therapist led part of her Bridges program. At that time, it was recommended that she retain her supervision hours for the next quarter so that the family could address strategies for any remaining (or new) inappropriate behaviors. It was also strongly recommended that future school placements not include adults who were aware of Molly's history, at least until she had established herself in the classroom. Molly seemed particularly susceptible to reducing her achievement to meet lowered expectations, and it was feared that she could take a very long time to overcome the effects of a teacher who did not hold her to the same standards as the rest of the class, even unintentionally.

Molly was very advanced academically and needed a class with many opportunities for interaction with peers with excellent language skills. It was suggested that as she matured she might be better suited for classes for gifted children. Molly now tolerated having people sing

Happy Birthday for other children at school and tolerated having it sung for her at school. She did not wish to have it sung for her at her home birthday party. As it did not seem appropriate to force Molly to endure Happy Birthday for her own birthday at home, she was allowed to choose a different song for her fourth birthday.

March 2005 (30 Months of ABA—End of the Program)

Molly had completed her Bridges program. Molly continued to function independently and to perform at both age and grade level in all environments. Her peer interactions at home and at school were consistent with those of typical children her age. Molly continued to attend school full time at a local private preschool for typically developing children. She had done well since her school support faded. Her teacher reported that Molly had continued to grow after her support faded. She had developed more mature peer relationships with several favored peers and accepted and initiated interactions with peers at a level comparable to that of her classmates. She displayed appropriate empathy and understanding of social cues in the school environment.

During the last months of observation, Molly consistently responded to enthusiasm from both adults and children. She was observed on at least one occasion to discern with no help what was funny about an incongruous story. She displayed social referencing skills and responded to body language and other nonvocal cues. Molly seemed happy to be at school with her friends. Observations at home and school showed that spontaneous language continued to be frequent and complex and to reflect appropriate awareness of the perspective of Molly's conversational partner. Behaviors were consistent with levels found in typical children.

Molly now seemed cheerful during classroom renditions of Happy Birthday.

June 2005 (3 Months After ABA)

I was able to see Molly again as I visited her class with a parent of another client observing various preschool options for her child. Molly was 4½ years old now. She played with other little girls in the class, talked to all of her classmates, and was at the top of her class academically. I had asked Molly's mother if I could mention her to the new parent and had been given permission. I asked the parent to pick out the child in the class with a history of autism. She could not—and this parent was experienced in the field.

Later that day I stood in the preschool hallway with tears in my eyes. Working with Molly had been a roller coaster ride from the very first day, and to see her there, happy and friendly and willing to do whatever anyone asked her to do, was something I had once thought we might never see.

Between June 2005 and February 2007

The family moved to another school district after Molly finished with us. Molly has no IEP. No teacher has suggested that she has any sort of problems. Molly was enrolled in kindergarten and started in September 2005, 3 months before her fifth birthday. Her kindergarten teacher was not told of her history until after she had been in the classroom for a while and was astonished when she was told. The parents have not told Molly's first-grade teacher of her history. The school administrators do not seem to be aware of it, either, though of course they are involved with her brother. At Molly's first-grade Christmas play, she was on stage with all of the first, second, and third graders. Molly danced for everyone!

February 2007 (2 Years After the Program Ended)

Molly's mom said this about her: "She is a perfect little wonderful angel—always singing. . . . I can't think of anything I would change about her."

She related this story:

Molly had always been afraid of her Uncle Ben's guitar and microphone. The extended family often had small "concerts" with Uncle Ben. There were many years when the family would pack up and leave to avoid a screaming tantrum from Molly. This year, Molly's brother sang a solo.

And so did Molly.

7

The Case of Nicholas B.

GLEN O. SALLOWS AND TAMLYNN D. GRAUPNER

Nick was the smaller of twin boys. He was born weighing 5 pounds, 1 ounce, and his brother weighed 6 pounds, 3 ounces. The pregnancy was followed closely because their mother was 36 years old and multiple births were involved. Mrs. B. had some spotting at 8 weeks' gestation and was put on medication to control preterm labor beginning at 6 months. She developed preeclampsia 3–4 weeks prior to the due date, and the twins were delivered at 36 weeks' gestation.

Nick's initial developmental milestones were within normal limits. He walked at 13 months and spoke his first word at 15 months. However, by 18 months, he had only five words and had stopped learning new ones. His parents took him to the pediatrician because they were concerned that he was not speaking more. Because Nick had had several ear infections, the pediatrician thought that perhaps he had a problem with his hearing. However, an audiologist found that his hearing was fine.

At home, the toddlers did little together, and Nick showed no interest in his twin brother, Evan. When outside, Evan would imitate their father as he worked in the yard, helping to move piles of mulch from one place to another. Nick, in contrast, would sit and sift the mulch through his fingers again and again, seemingly mesmerized by the activity. He did other unusual things in the yard, such as shaking bushes, feeling the bark on trees, and running his hands through the grass. Nick's parents became increasingly concerned as he began repetitively stacking blocks, toys, books, and cars, rather than using them for their intended purpose. They thought he understood some things, such as "Want a bath?," "Go car?," "Diaper," and "Laundry," but they could not be sure because Nick was inconsistent in his responses. They heard him say a couple of words, such as "ball" when he saw a hot air balloon and "bird," but there were few other times that Nick used words.

At about 21 months, Nick's brother, Evan, began showing rapid growth in language and gained approximately 200 words in the next 2 months. However, Nick did not learn any new words, and his parents took him to the doctor again. This time, at age 23 months, the pediatrician saw not just delays in language but also delays in social skills. Nick had poor eye contact, never approached his parents, and avoided them whenever they tried to interact with him. The doctor suspected autism and referred Nick's parents to an occupational therapist, a physical therapist, and a speech pathologist. He also referred them to the Wisconsin Early Autism Project for an evaluation.

The Screening

We first met Nick when he was 24 months old. Nick seemed unresponsive to our attempts to interest him in toys or in any kind of interaction. He did not smile or make eye contact. Whenever we tried to interact with him, he would leave. He did not understand gestures. For example, when I held my hand out for him to give me a block, he put it in a nearby container. I was surprised by this response and asked his mother about it. She explained that he had been dumping containers full of toys all over their playroom, so she had decided to teach him to clean up. It had taken months to get him to put things into a container, but she finally had gotten him to do it. Now, whenever he had something in his hand, he thought he was supposed to put it away.

Nick's language seemed quite delayed. During the screening, Nick did not speak, nor did he seem to understand verbal instructions. He could not name any familiar objects such as a car or spoon, nor did he respond when told, "sit down" or "come here."

Nick's play was unusual. He picked up toys and looked at them, but he did not play with them. Instead, when given several animal figurines, he held them up and slowly dropped them in front of his eyes or scrambled them around on the floor. He did the same thing with dollhouse furniture. When we brought out a simple puzzle, he did not understand what to do with it. He stacked the pieces and then began another stack 6 inches away. His father demonstrated how to make a car go on a track, but Nick got up and left. His mother tried to roughhouse with him by tickling him and laughing, but he tried to squirm away. When his father insisted that he sit in the chair, Nick began to whine.

As we discussed our observations and some of our concerns about Nick's behavior, his parents said that they had seen these behaviors at home but were unsure how to interpret them. Realizing that Nick was showing significant delays in language and social understanding, his mother grew tearful as she was confronted with the reality that something was very wrong with Nick.

Pretreatment Assessment

We conducted a battery of tests to evaluate Nick's cognitive, language, social, adaptive, and perceptual abilities. His cognitive abilities as measured on the Bayley Scales of Infant Development II were at 11 months when he was 24 months old, a 54% delay. Nick was not able to identify any familiar objects either by pointing to them or naming them. By dividing his mental ability (11 months) by his age (24 months), we estimated his IQ at 44, which is in the moderately mentally retarded range.

Nick's language skills were assessed using the Reynell Developmental Language Scales. This test utilizes many objects so that a child, who may not understand that pictures are the same as objects, can still give acceptable responses. The Reynell gives age equivalents as low as 12 months in receptive language and 15 months in expressive language. Nick's abilities were lower than could be measured in both areas, indicating severe language delays.

The Vineland Adaptive Behavior Scales is a widely used test that measures four adaptive domains: Communication in daily life, Daily Living Skills, Socialization, and Motor Skills. The test yields age equivalents as well as standard scores, where an "adequate" or average score ranges from 85 to 115. On the overall Adaptive Behavior Composite, Nick received a score of 64, with an age equivalent of 12 months, indicating "low functioning" and a 50% delay. On the individual domains, his Communication score was 64, with an age equivalent of 10 months (low); Daily Living Skills, including self-care, was 67, or 13 months (low); Socialization was 65, or 9 months (low); and Motor Skills was 81, or 18 months (moderately low). It is common for social and communication scores to be low in children with autism.

We also administered the Autism Diagnostic Interview-Revised (ADI-R), which at the time was the "gold standard" of diagnostic tools. Nick scored in the autistic range on all three scales, showing problems in communication, social skills, and idiosyncratic behavior.

Getting Started

We hired a team of three college students who were each scheduled to work three 2-hour shifts per week. Since Nick still napped, we began with two shifts per day and a total of 20 hours per week. The first therapist came from 8:30 AM to 10:30 AM Nick had lunch, and a second therapist worked with him from 12:30 PM to 2:30 PM, when Nick would be ready for a nap.

Nick's initial workshop was held in April 1997, when he was 28 months old. The senior therapist, three line therapists, myself, Nick, and his parents came together to learn how to implement the treatment program. We began in the morning, took hourly breaks, had lunch, and worked for about an hour in the afternoon. We taught Nick's parents and the student therapists to play with him so that he would be excited to see them when they arrived to work with him. We taught them to do each program from the curriculum that we were using and how to keep a record of Nick's responses. This information was kept in his "data book," which was a permanent record of what Nick had learned.

During the workshop, we started with easy and fun things in order to build a positive relationship with him. We played the "come here" game, in which the team stood in a circle and took turns calling Nick, saying "come here," while the person nearest Nick gave him a gentle nudge toward the caller to help him understand what he was supposed to do. Upon reaching the caller, Nick was given a hug and a small treat to make him happy that he had come. At first, Nick needed the nudge (physical guidance) to help him go to the person calling him. He wanted whatever treat the therapist had. Initially, he did not want hugs or tickles, but rather a bit of gummy worm, and gradually he went to the therapist without much help. After just 10–15 minutes of training, he came on his own when we said "come here."

We introduced simple tasks to convey the idea that what we wanted him to learn was easy and that he could succeed with a minimum of effort. The first tasks were "matching," putting a paper plate on top of another identical paper plate, and "nonverbal imitation," putting a ring from a ring-stacker toy on its pole, after we had demonstrated doing this. We chose these items because nesting items are easy to learn to match and because Nick's parents had told us that he already knew how to use the ring stacker. Initially, although he watched the demonstration, he did not understand that we wanted him to copy us. However, after we provided physical guidance a few times to show him how to pick up the plate and put it on the other one, he did it himself. Similarly, he put the ring on the pole after one prompt. Next, we modeled taking turns putting on the rings.

We helped Nick learn to follow verbal instructions by pairing them with a simple gesture. For example, we helped him learn what "give" meant by first giving him an object, then saying "give" while holding out our hand and tapping the object and then our open palm. Nick needed physical guidance a few times, such as our moving his hand toward our open palm, but he quickly got the idea.

We also introduced a large knob puzzle, in which all the pieces were separate and each piece matched a picture in an opening. He dumped all the pieces out and began stacking them into piles instead of putting them into the puzzle board. We decided to take out just one piece and physically guide him to put it back in without playing with it. He learned this after two or three tries, or "trials." We "reinforced" or rewarded Nick after each of his attempts to pair the idea of his focusing on a task and following our nonverbal instructions (the demonstrations) with something positive. Nick became more interested and happy to participate.

After every three or four trials (e.g., placing the paper plate three times, which took about 30 seconds), we would say "Go play" and would attempt to join Nick in play on the floor. This was difficult at first because Nick disliked having other people try to interact with him. As therapists tried to get him to play with toys appropriately, Nick became somewhat upset because he enjoyed playing in his own repetitive and self-stimulatory way. We had to be careful not to "ruin" his fun. We stayed nearby and played with Nick in parallel, much the way toddlers play near each other, without touching his toys or directing him to do anything differently. After a few days, Nick became less concerned when we were nearby or wanted to join him in play.

During each hour with Nick, the therapists would present an activity such as matching, imitating actions, following instructions, or doing puzzles for 30–60 seconds and then play with him for a few minutes. Over the course of an hour, Nick was presented with each activity numerous times, allowing him so much practice and success that he learned new skills at quite a fast rate. After working in this fashion for about 45 minutes, the therapist and Nick would take a 15-minute break, perhaps going outside to the swing or for a walk.

Nick's therapists were trained to implement each program, first watching as the senior therapist demonstrated, then taking turns implementing the activity with Nick. Because there were only a few activities to learn, the therapists as well as Nick's parents learned the programs within a few turns. In addition to learning how to implement the activities, the therapists learned the positive style of interaction that we used while working and playing with Nick. They learned to be "reinforcing" by practicing how to get Nick to smile or laugh; to use short phrases when speaking, because Nick did not understand much language; and to reward Nick for trying our activities, because he often preferred to do things his way.

Each therapist received 30 hours of training, including 10–15 hours of supervised one-on-one work with Nick before they worked with him alone. We used a checklist of the skills the therapists needed to learn, and they were trained in each skill. We taught them to observe closely and record whether Nick did activities correctly so that we could modify the program on an ongoing basis to help him learn as fast as he was able. We also taught the therapists to always be aware of Nick's emotional response to treatment and to adjust the tasks and their interactions with him to keep him successful and happy so that he would remain motivated to keep learning.

We held a team meeting with Nick, his parents, and all of his therapists every week. During these meetings, Nick's parents presented information on how he was doing at home, and the therapists discussed and demonstrated each program so that everybody could agree and become more consistent in their work with Nick. On the basis of this information, we introduced and demonstrated new programs, which everybody practiced with Nick until they could implement each program correctly. If Nick had problems at home or with learning a skill, we discussed troubleshooting strategies and developed alternate programming to address the problem or teach the skill.

One Month After Treatment

Nick had learned to match 12 objects, and he could follow seven instructions. These were "come here," "sit," "high-five," "pick up," "stand up," "give," and "go play." Gestural cues were used with the verbal instructions, such as tapping the chair as we said "sit." He could imitate movements such as putting rings on a ring stacker, putting a block in a bucket, pounding on a drum, and stacking blocks. He could also do a 4 piece peg puzzle. He tended to want to stack the puzzle pieces, but we corrected this by prompting him to put the pieces into the puzzle without playing with them and rewarding him as soon as he had completed the task. He would look up at us and smile when we cheered for him after a success. He seemed proud that he could do so many things, and he was excited about how happy his mother and father were. After days filled with activity and the undivided attention of the therapists, Nick began to sleep better at night, was generally happier, and loved to have his therapists come every day. His babbling had increased, and he was beginning to make approximations of words as we said them.

Although Nick's team had received training to implement the first steps of his program, they were still fairly inexperienced and made some mistakes. For instance, while the senior therapist and I were away for a few days, the team continued to have Nick match the same 12 items, long after he could do them easily. Nick became restless and whined when he saw the therapist preparing to do the matching program. We addressed this by introducing new matching items and by clarifying the guidelines for therapists, so they would know when an item was learned and when to introduce new items.

Another mistake occurred in the receptive instruction program. The team tried to teach him to wave and say "bye-bye" when they gave the instruction "wave bye-bye." This was too difficult because Nick was not yet able to speak reliably, even though he would occasionally try to imitate a word. He would have to learn to imitate many more sounds and words before the team could expect him to say "bye-bye" when asked.

Three Months After Treatment

When Nick was 2 years, 6 months old, we increased his weekly hours to 25. He had made many gains. He could do a 9-piece peg puzzle the first time he saw it. He could match complex picture cards, imitate seven gestures, and follow eight instructions such as "come here" without any cues or prompts. Language was increasing rapidly. He could identify 50 objects receptively; that is, upon hearing the label, he could find the right item. He could also say approximations of 10 object names. If he had trouble with one item, we would stop that one and try another, coming back to the harder one when he had gained more skill by working on other items.

We also began an "interactive play" program to directly address Nick's ability to respond to our initiations and to allow us to join him. Playing interactively requires a complex set of skills, and we taught therapists each skill. They had to learn how to keep his interest high, to follow his lead at times, and, most important, to watch Nick's nonverbal responses closely so that they could modify their initiations to avoid overwhelming his readiness to accept their social approaches. One goal was to teach therapists to approach and play with Nick in such a way that he would not turn away or leave. Once a therapist could do this, he or she could gradually begin to address interactive play goals such as learning appropriate toy play and responding to other's initiations through joining and encouraging Nick to stay focused on a theme. These were all skills that Nick would need in order to successfully play with other children. It was much easier for him to learn these skills first in a friendly relationship with a trusted adult, who was tolerant of social errors and could repair communication breakdowns.

In their desire to help Nick make more progress, the team had been pressing him to stay on task for 20–30 minutes at a time. Nick seemed to be getting fatigued and less cooperative. During the early phases of treatment, our usual goal for sustained attention is a few minutes at a time. We wanted Nick's on-task time to be as positive as possible so that he would be happy to return to work. Though he could be pressed to work longer, he had begun to feel less motivated and to act as if he disliked the activities. Therefore, we had the team shorten the intervals of work while inserting more play time.

After 3 months of treatment, Nick's parents took him back to the developmental pediatrician to get his opinion on how he was doing. The doctor noted that Nick spontaneously labeled "cat" when he was looking at a book, and he took the book to his dad to have it read to him (a spontaneous social initiation!). He also sang a song using about 50% intelligible words. The doctor commented that "the most striking change in Nick was his significant amount of forward progress."

Nick had been doing quite well, but then he began having difficulty with imitation and following directions, activities with which he had previously been quite successful. His mother hypothesized that he was bored and needed new material, and it is true that novelty often increases attention. The team therefore added many new items. In nonverbal imitation, Nick had learned to imitate seven movements and the team had introduced five new ones at once. In receptive instructions (following verbal instructions), Nick understood eight, and the team had introduced six more at once. Unfortunately, Nick became overwhelmed with so many new things to learn at the same time and began "scrolling." That is, he would run through all of the new responses, hoping that one of them was correct. This problem can lead to confusion regarding already learned material, so it was important to remedy the problem quickly. Although Nick was losing interest in these two activities, he was happy during other programs, indicating that he still felt generally successful. Fortunately, we caught this error quickly enough and reduced the number of new items he was working on in time to avoid his discouragement with the two programs from spreading to other programs or therapy in general.

As Nick learned more language, we began to focus on generalizing his ability to apply a label to any object in the environment in response to any question. We took Nick with us around the house and yard to be sure he could identify a tree or a stove, for example, in response to several question forms such as "Where is the ball?" or "Can you find the car?," "What's that?," or "Show me the spoon." Nick was also beginning to use speech spontaneously outside therapy with other people.

After 5 months of treatment, at age 2 years, 5 months, Nick occasionally used a poorly articulated two-word phrase to request (e.g., "Green ball?"), and he could easily label the colors on a multicolored object. However, his interest in animal cards was getting to be an obsession, and he wanted them all the time. He had begun to sift them through his fingers, watching them drop to the floor. We had to restrict Nick's access to the cards and finally to "lose them." We taught him more interactive games that he could use with peers, such as shooting baskets, having pillow fights, and playing Pop Up Pirates.

Six Months After Treatment

At about this time, Nick's parents enrolled him in a preschool 2 days per week, 4 hours per day. One of his therapists went to school to work with him for 1 hour on each of the 2 days. We had recommended that Nick not be enrolled in preschool because his spontaneous language was still rudimentary. He had many single-word labels, but he could not converse, and although he had learned to play appropriately with several toys, he had little experience interacting with peers. We decided to observe Nick at school after several weeks there to see how he was doing and then report back to his parents.

Six weeks later, when we arrived at Nick's classroom, the teacher was reading a story to the children. All the children except Nick were sitting quietly listening to the story. One of the teachers was trying to hold him on her lap, talking to him, hoping to redirect his attention to the story. Nick, however, was struggling to get down, and the more the teacher held him, the harder he struggled. Eventually, he began to whine and yell. He was disrupting everybody in the class, so the teacher had to remove him.

A few minutes later, it was time to go outside to the playground. Nick walked around by himself, seeming to explore the yard, but he didn't play with anything. He did not approach any children or talk to anyone. Similarly, none of the children approached him or tried to talk to him. We did a formal observation, logging the number of times that he approached someone or anybody approached him. During the next 40 minutes, the number of social interactions was 1, but when the child approached, Nick did not acknowledge him and walked away.

When we reported this information back to his parents, they were quite surprised because the preschool staff had felt that Nick was adjusting well to the classroom. Our observation showed that in fact Nick was not yet ready to learn from group experiences. Nick's parents decided to remove him from preschool because he was spending many hours per week at school but interacting little, when he could be at home learning skills more quickly, including how to interact with his therapists, parents, brother, and neighbor children.

As the weeks of therapy continued, Nick learned to imitate consonant-vowel-consonant words (CVC) such as "Bob" and CVCV words such as "Bobby," moving from approximations of the words to articulating them perfectly. We then moved on to short phrases. He had learned animal sounds and names of rooms of the house, and he was learning to say the names of objects as quickly as we taught them to him. He continued to use one- and two-word phrases to request or to comment on things he saw. We decided to introduce sight reading because he was interested in books, and we thought that it might help him speak in longer phrases if he could read the phrase first.

After 9 Months of Treatment

At age 3 years, 1 month, Nick could count up to six objects on the table correctly. The strategy that finally worked for him was pushing down a lid on a pop-up toy for every number that he counted. This helped him understand that each number stood for a separate thing. Nick could also spell and read 15 words. We taught this by having him match individual letters to the letters in a printed word on a card that included a picture of the object. He would match the letters while saying each one. Once all the letters of the word were matched, we would say the whole word, and then he would say it. After doing this with several words, Nick began to say the letters and read the word on his own.

Nick thoroughly enjoyed interactive play with his therapists. He began to pretend to drink out of imaginary cups and eat with imaginary spoons at a tea party, and he thought it was funny when therapists or his brother did something silly. Nick was beginning to use what he had learned in therapy with other people in typical, novel situations. Nick's skills seemed to have become more integrated and easier for him to use.

After 10 months of treatment, at age 3 years, 2 months, Nick's parents wanted to devote more time to peer play, which we had been advocating for some time. His mom also began working with him 1 hour per day. This was an important step for her because it meant that she would become much more knowledgeable about how he learned. It would also allow her to make more useful suggestions to the team.

Nick could follow 31 verbal instructions such as "get your coat" and "bring me my shoes." He could sort different types of items by category and count objects with 1:1 correspondence. He was doing 21-piece jigsaw puzzles and enjoyed them just for fun. He could read 23 sight words and some short phrases. We had begun to teach him prepositions, including "on top," "inside," "outside," and "under," and Nick was able to learn them easily.

After 1 Year of Treatment

Nick had completed his first year of treatment at age 39½ months, and we repeated the battery of tests to examine his progress. On the Bayley II, his age equivalent was 37–39 months, and his Mental Development

Index (IQ) was 103, solidly in the average range. On the Reynell language test, his receptive language age equivalent was 28 months (up from under 12 months), and his expressive language age equivalent was 26 months (up from under 15 months), yielding standard scores of 65 and 63, respectively. While his age equivalents were significantly higher than Nick had shown prior to beginning therapy, his language was still quite delayed. At 39½ months old, he was 11 months behind his age mates in understanding language, a 28% delay, and 13 months behind in expressive language, a 33% delay. Regarding adaptive functioning, Nick received an Adaptive Behavior Composite score on the Vineland of 69, with an age equivalent of 25 months (up from 12 months), showing a delay of 14 months, or 36%, in comparison to other children his age. The largest gain Nick made in adaptive skills was in the Communication domain, with a standard score of 92 and an age equivalent of 34 months, well within the average range for a child Nick's age.

During the second year of treatment, we increased his therapy time to 30 hours per week. This included weekly peer play with his brother and a child from the neighborhood, beginning with just one session per week. Nick had already learned to play interactively with us using many different kinds of toys. During the first several play dates, the goal was to have the children enjoy being together. We introduced interactive games that required minimal speech, such as Duck-Duck-Goose, Ring Around the Rosy, chase, and Hide and Seek. We also included simple table-top games that involved a lot of action, such as Hungry Hungry Hippo, Lucky Ducks, Pop Up Pirates, and Don't Break the Ice. The team also wanted to use bean bags in simple tossing games.

During the first several weeks of peer-play sessions, Nick had a tendency to be bossy and unwilling to do activities that the other child wanted to do. He would want to leave and play alone. Nick also got upset if he lost a game. We helped Nick to become more flexible by working with him one-on-one with no children present. We had the therapists pretend they needed help or act as if they had made a mistake and ask Nick for help to boost his self-esteem. We accidentally knocked over our towers and asked Nick for help in rebuilding the tower. We said we wanted a toy that Nick was holding and asked him to trade with us. We convinced Nick that it was fair to take turns selecting the next activity and coaxed him to play with us, even when it was not his favorite game. Since we were familiar to Nick, he was more willing to go along with what we wanted and to let us have toys that he would usually not want to share. We practiced these skills and used Social Stories and Video Modeling to help Nick understand how his playmates felt when he would not play with them. We also used these strategies to show Nick how to interact with playmates so that they would have fun and want to play with him. We then helped him generalize his social learning to peer-play sessions.

We taught Nick self-care activities such as washing hands, brushing teeth, dressing, and sitting at the table to eat. We taught him to stay in the yard by placing cones around the perimeter of the yard and explaining to him that he was supposed to stay within the cones. If he left the yard, he had to come inside for a few minutes. Both Nick and Evan quickly learned the concept and every other cone was removed; soon only every third cone remained, until there were no cones left and the boys consistently stayed in their own yard.

At age 3 years, 5 months, Nick was still not toilet trained. He did not like messy diapers and would say, "I want a clean fresh one." We planned a "Big Day" where Nick would have a fun day practicing to use the potty. To make it more likely that Nick would need to use the toilet, he got to have as much juice as he wanted. Each time he used the potty, Nick got a special reward of his favorite treat, strawberry ice cream. Nick wore big-boy underpants that he had picked out himself, and within that day Nick learned to use the toilet. He had proven to himself that going on the potty was something he knew how to do, and he was mostly successful from then on. He had a habit of beginning to take his pants off while he was running to the bathroom, and we had to address this because he did it at school as well.

Nick was also not interested in dressing himself. We had not yet worked on this, as reflected in his low score on self-care in testing. He would not even put on a swimming suit to go swimming because he enjoyed being helped. We decided to use the strategy of having Nick choose which items of clothing he wanted to put on. The therapist would ask him, "What do you want to put on first?" and let him choose. He could choose what to wear and when to put it on. We also used Video Modeling to show Evan and Nick getting dressed so that they could watch together. This served to build general interest in the activity of dressing for both boys. They thought it was fun to see themselves on TV.

Nick could now identify emotions displayed by the therapists, his parents, and Evan, and he could describe the actions as we demonstrated them. He would say, for instance, "You are jumping," "Ben is reading." Because Nick was able to use sentences now, we began the "statement-statement" program, in which Nick learned to speak back and forth with the therapists. The therapist would say "I have a jelly sandwich" and another person responded by saying, "I have a bologna sandwich." With a little prompting, Nick quickly caught on to this new skill and began using it around the house. We taught Nick when to use many kinds of questions, such as "What is it?," when we said we had a surprise for him or "Where is it?" when he could not find something. One strategy that we used was to play a game of hiding an animal from his animal basket. He knew exactly which one was missing, and, after prompting him to ask "Where is the tiger?" we told him where it was.

When we first tried to teach Nick to say, "What?" when someone called his name, he responded by imitating what we had said, that is, he would say, "Say what." We were able to teach this skill by remaining silent as we showed him a word card with "What?" printed on it after calling his name. We also decided to introduce the "yes and no" program. He could answer correctly for factual questions; for example, if you asked him "Is this a tiger?" and it was really an elephant, he would say, "No, it's an elephant." We wanted to teach him to answer "yes" or "no" with regard to things offered to him because this would be a useful skill in real life. We held a glass of juice up and asked him, "Do you want some juice?" then prompted him to say "Yes." When he learned to do this, we offered something he did not like, asked him if he wanted it, and prompted him to say "No." This was a little difficult for him and took several weeks to learn.

After 18 Months of Treatment

At 3 years, 9 months old, we increased Nick's hours to 36 per week, including 7 hours per week of peer play. He was re-enrolled in pre-school. His adjustment went well, and the teachers felt he was doing fine. A therapist attended for an hour each day, primarily to watch for social problems, which we then addressed at home. She noticed that Nick did not seem to stand up for himself when children took his things, whereas his brother would say, "No, I need that." We taught Nick to say the same thing using Video Modeling and practicing with us and with peers.

Nick could play with us and with neighbor children one at a time, but at school, Nick still seemed largely indifferent toward the other children and was not "socializing." Nick knew a few of their names, and he tolerated their presence when they approached to play near him, but he did not interact much. When the therapist tried to encourage Nick to play with the other children, he said, "No, thank you." From previous experience, we knew that it would work better if Nick was approached by other children in activities that he was already doing. Therefore, our shadow started a game that Nick liked, "What's the time, Mr. Fox?" Before long, several other children came to join. We also had Nick's mother invite children from preschool to come home for play dates.

At home, several therapists noted that if they were next to him, Nick would respond appropriately when spoken to, but if he was engaged in an activity and was perhaps 10–15 feet away, he did not respond. We decided that this was an important skill to target. With a therapist near him, another called him from farther away. We showed him how to answer by raising our voice and saying, "What?"

The team was doing well with developing strategies for dealing with problems the family had with Nick in everyday life and with coming up with ways to teach Nick new skills. The team did well with arranging for a shadow in school and during peer play at home. When asked how much time they spent working with Nick, his parents were unable to be specific but said it was virtually all the time.

Because many children with autism do not learn much prior to treatment, they have missed out on a lot of "cultural knowledge." To help them be able to interact with peers, it is important that they know things that other children their age know. As an example, we taught "occupations" so that Nick learned what different people did for work. For instance, we would ask, "Who likes to cook food?" and he knew that it was a cook or a chef. We also introduced him to currently popular toys such as Power Rangers and suggested that his parents have him watch the TV shows.

Nick also did the "drawing" program in which he learned to hold a pencil, copy shapes, draw dot to dots, make letters and numbers, and draw pictures of objects such as houses and trees. He learned to do some beginning negotiating by agreeing to do an activity that another person wanted to do and then saying, "And then we can do what I want to do."

We used the "telling a story" program as another way to increase language and spontaneous speech. Nick and the therapist used a felt board, placing animals and other items on the board as they alternated making up a sentence about what the animals were doing. Nick got involved in the story and wanted to add more sentences to help decide how it was going to end. The therapists also used this activity to work with other concepts such as past tense and pronouns.

After 2 Years of Treatment

Nick was tested again in April 1999, at age 4 years, 5 months. He was tested by a local community psychologist unaffiliated with WEAP. She used the WPPSI-R IQ test, the Vineland Adaptive Behavior Scales, and one part of the Woodcock-Johnson III Tests of Achievement, Broad Reading. On the WPPSI-R, Nick achieved a Performance IQ Score of 87, a Verbal IQ Score of 100, and a Full-Scale IQ Score of 94, essentially in the average range. He scored high on object assembly (puzzles), vocabulary, and similarities, reflecting his advanced understanding of puzzles and words, and he was above average on information (general knowledge). His low scores were in mazes and arithmetic, reflecting the fact that we had not worked much on writing or arithmetic. He also had a low score in comprehension, reflecting a problem with thinking about the right thing to do in an unfamiliar situation, a common problem for children with autism.

On the Vineland Adaptive Behavior Scales, his overall standard score was 73. This represented improvement but also indicated continued delay in comparison to other children his age. In Communication, a measure of everyday language, Nick scored 124, in the superior range, but his score on Socialization was 71, reflecting his continuing social difficulties. On the Woodcock-Johnson, Nick received a Broad Reading age percentile of 99.9, showing that he could read better than almost all children his age.

In September 1999, when Nick was 4 years, 9 months old, he was attending preschool every morning and public school in the afternoon for 2 half-days per week. We reduced his therapy time at home to 15 hours per week. When I observed Nick at school, he seemed happy, greeted me, and told me what he was doing on the computer. A child approached him, seeming interested in what he was talking about, but Nick rebuffed him a little too assertively. Nick wanted to tell me more about his work and seemed worried that the other child was going to interfere.

At this early point in the school term, Nick was still adjusting and clearly needed his therapist and teacher to help him interact appropriately with other children. We decided to use Video Modeling to demonstrate how to invite others who approached to join him and how to negotiate when a child wanted to take something Nick was still using.

We checked in at school regularly to monitor how Nick was doing and offered advice for troubleshooting problems as they arose. When I saw him a month later, he was talking with several children, but he talked more with adults. Nick did fine if an adult got things started, but he was still reluctant to initiate contact with peers.

We began talking with Nick's parents about his remaining social goals, which included joining others and telling peers where he was going when he decided to leave. Frequently at school, he would leave play unannounced, wandering off and leaving the other child wondering what had happened and why Nick had walked away. Once, when asked why he had left, he said, "I changed my mind. I made another choice." We taught Nick to look at the person he was with, get the person's attention, and say something like, "I'm done playing. I'm going to the blocks." Teaching him the skills he needed to join others was a little more complex. We decided that he needed to learn how to observe what other children were doing, generate ideas about what he might do with them, and know what to say to join them.

In therapy at home, we focused on each skill in turn. We wrote social stories about looking around the classroom and describing what the children were doing. We practiced with Nick at school, and, with the help of his shadow, he became comfortable with looking around the room and choosing where he would like to play. The next objective was to help Nick learn what to do as he tried to join a group of children that he wanted to play with. It was a little painful to watch Nick repeatedly try unsuccessfully to join a group when the other children could not hear him because he spoke too softly or when they did not invite him to play. He needed to develop a repertoire of skills with which to manage being rebuffed. He also needed to learn how to act to make it more likely that children would invite him to join their play.

We went to our own 5-year-old's preschool classroom and watched what our son, Neil, did as he entered the room first thing in the morning. He had already developed the strategy of surveying the children and selecting the activity he was interested in joining. As Neil approached a couple of boys who were running cars on a track, he said, "Hi, can I play?" One of the boys said, without looking up,

"No. We only have enough cars for us." Neil stood for a moment and then announced to the boys, "I hurt my eye." One boy looked up with interest and said, "I hurt my arm," showing his bandage. Neil sat down near the boys and reached for a car that was not in use and put it on the track as the second boy said, "Let me see your eye." A conversation about bodily injury ensued as the three boys played with their cars.

We were surprised to see that Neil's tactic had worked. We made notes about how other children behaved in order to join groups, and some were helpful. One boy just approached a group, commented, "I'll be the red one," and sat down to join the car race. We made several videos showing ways that children joined groups for Nick to watch and practice. In the end, though, it just happened by chance. At preschool, a girl joined him as he played with dinosaurs. Nick was making a "dinosaur museum" and let her place a few dinos in the museum. She then started feeding them, which Nick objected to, saying, "They're just bones, so we shouldn't feed them," but he allowed her to feed a few, anyway. After a few minutes, she shifted her interest to a doll-house that was nearby, and Nick joined her, bringing a container with more people in it, and they played together for some time.

After 3 Years of Treatment

Nick was tested again by an outside psychologist. He was 5 years, 4 months old on the day of his testing. On the WPSSI-R, he achieved a Full Scale IQ of 109. His Verbal IQ Score was 112, and his Performance IQ was 104, all in the average range. On the Reynell language scale, Nick's standard scores were 106 in Verbal Comprehension and 80 in Expressive Language, both showing large improvements in comparison to his scores during the first 2 years. His language skills had improved significantly because of the combined effect of learning conversational skills in therapy and his many hours at school and in peer play where we had helped him to use language in typical settings. On the Vineland, Nick's composite score was 73, still moderately low, while Communication remained high at 116. In other areas, Nick continued to hold his place relative to peers, but he was not closing the gap.

Nick was scheduled to begin kindergarten in the fall. His parents decided to start a playgroup in their basement for children in the neighborhood who were going to attend kindergarten with Nick. They sent out letters to local families and got responses from several. The group was 90 minutes long and was scheduled once per week. It was structured so that new activities were introduced every 5–10 minutes. We had one therapist for every two children so that any child needing help got it quickly and most potential difficulties could be resolved before anybody got upset. Happily, Nick was invited to a birthday party soon after the group began. Nick and Evan joined a gymnastics class, and both did well. The instructors were unaware that Nick had been diagnosed with autism.

Kindergarten

When school began, in the fall, Nick's parents decided to inform the school that he had been diagnosed with autism, that he was high functioning, but that he still struggled in some situations. He did not have a shadow or an aide. Nick's teacher wrote a note each day about how things had gone and sent it home with Nick for his parents and therapists to read and use as a guide for goals in therapy.

Nick had begun to function in much the same way as other children his age, although he was still somewhat controlling. Once at morning circle, the teacher was preparing to read a book to the children when Nick stood up and said, "I don't like that book. I want this book," as he held his up. The teacher handled this perfectly when she told him that she had already picked a book but that she could read his book another day. He accepted this without protest and sat down.

A few weeks into the term, Nick became upset when he saw two children fighting on the playground. He said, "I hate those kids." We thought that he might have been frightened by the fight and wanted to help him understand what had happened. We explained that a fight can start when someone makes a mistake and another person gets angry. Nick seemed to understand, but he still felt it was wrong.

We were concerned that Nick might make other children angry by not understanding playground rules, so we discussed the fact that there were rules that children needed to follow, for example, not climbing up the slide backward. We also explained that teachers were there to help children when they were having trouble, and he became comfortable with the idea that the teacher would take care of things. In the classroom, Nick began to notice when other children were misbehaving and started telling the other children that they were not following the rules. We had to clarify for him that the teacher was in charge in the classroom and that she would take care of things. Since Nick was in school full time, his hours of therapy at home were reduced to about 10 hours per week, most of which addressed social issues. His parents commented that he seemed more interested in others.

After Nick entered first grade in a regular classroom, I observed him after he had been in the room for about a month. He sat with the rest of the class listening to the teacher. When it was time to clean up, Nick did so willingly. However, when recess time came, Nick said, "I don't want to go out." The teacher told him that it was not a choice and he said, "Okay." We had suggested that the teacher use this phrase after we had worked with Nick to help him understand the idea that some things were a choice, but other things, like following the teacher's instructions, were not a choice.

The teacher had little experience with autism and had some trouble understanding how to deal with Nick, who had been taking markers and other items off of her desk. She was allowing the classroom aide to help him but had not interacted with him herself. We suggested that she get to know him by working with him herself. Afterward, she found Nick was much more responsive to her and commented that she now understood him. She said, "He's really not a problem in class," jokingly asking if we could help her with another child.

At recess, Nick and a small group of children played together, taking turns demonstrating their trick ways of bouncing a ball. As the weeks moved on and we checked in with his teacher, she said that she had been able to handle any problems with Nick by making rules with him about doing things when it was time, completing his work projects before he began to do another activity, and staying with the group.

Nick was chosen for the Talented and Gifted program, and he went to a session while I was there. He was in a room with seven other kindergarteners and first graders, and they were going to do a play. First they listened to the teacher read the play, and then they were supposed to each pick a part. Nick picked a part but then quickly changed his mind. The teacher told him that she would have to come back to him. This did not seem to bother him much, although he reminded her a few times not to forget. When she got to him again, he said he wanted to be the fox. Then two other children also picked the part of the fox, so there were three children who wanted to be the fox. After everyone had picked a part, the teacher presented the problem to the group. They had three foxes, but no chickens. She asked the class what they thought should be done. There was silence. Nobody had an idea. Then, to my great and pleasant surprise, Nick volunteered to be the chicken, even though the fox was clearly a higher status role in the play. This was the first time I had seen Nick make a decision to give up something he wanted for the greater good of the group.

Outside on the playground, he was with a group of children. It was difficult to hear what they were saying, but they seemed to be pretending they were all running from a monster. He was with this group for the entire recess. I noticed that he seemed to be poking fun and teasing a child that he disliked. It almost seemed like he was doing it for attention or approval from his peers. He said, "Look, it's Malcolm. Oh no!" The fact that he seemed to be aware of his peer's probable reaction (evidence of "theory of mind") was a great advance in social understanding, but we decided we should talk to him about the difference between being mean and being funny. Even so, his behavior was not that abnormal, and on that day, nobody would have picked Nick out as being any different from the other children.

Nick was tested after 4 years of treatment at age 6 years, 5 months. Verbal IQ was 132, Performance IQ was 99, and Full-Scale IQ was 118. Nick's teacher completed the Vineland. Nick received a 114 in Communication and a 92 in Socialization. On the Woodcock-Johnson III Tests of Achievement, Nick received scores of 122 in expressive language, 111 in comprehension, 121 in reading, 127 in matching, and 127 in academic abilities.

We asked his teacher to complete the Child Behavior Checklist (CBC), in which she looked over a large range of problem behaviors and checked those she felt were true of Nick. The CBC uses T scores, with an average range from 50 to 67. Scores from 67 to 70 are in the borderline problem range, and scores of 70 and above indicate clinically significant problems. The CBC has several scales (Withdrawn, Anxious/Depressed, Social Problems, Attention Problems, Aggression), and Nick scored in the "normal" range on all scales but Thought Problems, where he was in the borderline range. This scale, which reflects odd thought and preoccupations, was 69. The teacher rated him in the borderline range because of his long-standing interest in dinosaurs. Although Nick still liked them, he had also begun to develop many other interests from interacting with other children who liked to talk about and do things that were new to him.

We had a meeting with Nick's mother, and she said that all reports from school were positive. We thought it had helped that the teacher had formed a relationship with Nick. At home, he had made up an imaginary school with students and a name for the school. He was writing stories about his school. On the computer at home, he was doing academic programs such as Reader Rabbit and Jump Start Second Grade. For the first time, Nick also had a best friend, Caroline. The two of them were constant companions at school, and Nick got in trouble (delightfully) for talking too much in class. During the summer of that year, Nick was in a theater group, and he said that he liked acting. He was more interested in seeking out new friends and sharing his ideas.

In September, Nick started second grade. He did well at home, and his parents were pleased that he was talking to them about what was happening at school and asking questions about what was socially appropriate. A couple of months into second grade, Nick began to have some difficulty at school with being bullied. He had trouble telling the difference between friendly teasing and mean behavior. His parents talked with him about this and recommended that he stay away from those children or tell the teacher if they continued to bother him. They got children's books about how to be a good friend, and we coached his parents when they asked for advice. At this point, Nick's parents felt that they knew what to do about Nick's day-to-day issues, and they were ready to discontinue treatment.

Nick is now 13 years old and is in the eighth grade. His parents report that both boys are doing fine and do not remember much about the therapy years. Schoolwork is easy for Nick, and for the most part he is "moving along with the crowd." We've been in touch recently to arrange testing again, and his father expressed an interest in setting up outpatient counseling for Nick, mainly to address some anxiety about going into high school next year. We have counseled other children in their early teens over similar issues and have seen them move ahead and succeed without further services.

8

A Parent's Story: Jake and Nick

JUSTIN LEAF, RONALD LEAF, AND JAMISON DAYHARSH LEAF

Unless someone has had a child with autistic disorder, it is impossible to understand the pressures that mothers and fathers of such children feel. Starting with the diagnostic process, having to sort out the hundreds of treatment options, then having to deal with professionals with differing opinions (and who sometimes can be quite condescending) can be infuriating, devastating, and depressing.

Historically, parents have had to deal with tremendous guilt when they have a child with autism. They often ponder many questions about their lives, day after day. Were they responsible for their child's disorder? Did they do something wrong during pregnancy? Did they make the wrong decision regarding the birthing method? Did they not bond with their child? In the early days (see Chapter 7 for details), most professionals believed that the parents were responsible for their child's disorder.[1] Many professionals pointed to the parents as the culprit.

In addition to dealing with the anguish and perhaps guilt of having a child with a severe disability, parents immediately face a concomitant stress in their life. It will be their responsibility to get their child much-needed treatment. Typically, their lives are consumed with therapies. Their regimen can include driving to speech therapy and occupational therapy, opening up their home to have therapists tromp in at all hours, getting their child ready for school, attending clinics, and visiting the psychologist for the hopeful and sometimes dreaded reevaluation. In addition to the management of scheduled therapy and appointments, they must become experts in the treatment methodologies. It is not surprising or unrealistic for parents to feel that their child's entire existence and quality of life rests solely on their shoulders. What an absolutely incredible burden!

It is not surprising that parents become totally consumed and all too often feel they have no choice other than to sacrifice their lives and therefore their families' lives for the good of the child with autism. It is understandable that parents would make the ultimate sacrifice and do everything in their power to rescue their child with tremendous needs, their loved one. Clearly, if not for the family, the children would not have the opportunities for improvement. They would not have the support and nurturing to survive the challenges. It is ultimately the family that makes it happen!

Imagine the added stress of having two children with autism. If it were not for Grace and Todd, the parents of the children described in this chapter, we would not be able to share their family's triumph!

Jake's Story

As the alarm rings, Jake wakes from his deep sleep and thinks to himself, "It's just too early to get up, I just need 10 more minutes." Like most teenagers, Jake rolls over, hits the snooze button, and goes back to sleep. Thirty minutes later, Jake reluctantly rolls out of bed, hops into the shower, and gets ready for the day. After a quick breakfast, Jake is off to school. As he leaves the house, his mother tells him that he needs to come directly home after school because he has sailing practice. He hops on his bike and rides to Nobel Middle School.

Walking through the halls, Jake can think only about all the great things that the summer will bring—there is the family vacation to Washington, D.C., and time for riding his bike with his friends, swimming at the beach, Junior Guards, and his favorite activity, sailing. As Jake continues to walk through the halls, he spots a group of his closest friends and decides to join them before math class begins. The conversation is the same as on all other days—talk about the latest movies, which teachers they currently do not like, which girls they think are cute, and summer plans. As Jake is talking, another alarm rings, only this one tells him that he must hurry up and get to class. Over the next 6 hours Jake goes to and from class. Jake is in the Gifted and Talented Education (GATE) program and begins by going to math, then science, history, orchestra class, where he plays the clarinet, and finally football. While in class, Jake is usually paying attention to the teacher, but there are times when he daydreams instead. When the final bell rings, indicating that school is over, Jake races home for a quick snack and then is off to sailing practice. The rest of the night is filled with his regular routine—come home from practice, do homework, eat dinner with the family, and then play video games, sometimes with his younger brother, Nick.

Jake's story is like that of so many other eighth-grade boys. However, Jake is not like any average teenager. When Jake was 4 years old, he was diagnosed with Autistic Disorder (*DSM-IV* 299.00). Fortunately for Jake and his family, he has been able to achieve what many people would consider a miracle. It is what researchers have described as obtaining "best outcome," which is defined as not needing supports at school and being indistinguishable from other teens to his peers, his teachers, and others in the community. And, most important, Jake is happy! He is excelling at school, has a good group of friends, and has a bright outlook for the future. Though Jake has reached "best-outcome" status, his path has not been easy. It has taken a great deal of hard work from professionals, from his parents, and, most important, from Jake himself. This is Jake's story.

Prediagnosis and Diagnosis

In the spring of 1991, Grace and Todd were awaiting the arrival of their first child. Finally, after 9 months of an uneventful pregnancy, Jake came into the world, a beautiful 8 pound, 9 ounce boy. There was fetal distress during delivery, and an emergency cesarean section was performed. The return home was delayed until the 4th day because Jake needed to stay for observation due to cardiac arrhythmia. However, the next few months were filled with happiness and joy for Jake and his family. At 6 months of age, Jake was able to sit by himself; at 14 months, he was able to walk independently. A few months after that, Jake began saying single words. Grace and Todd were loving parents. They had a healthy, beautiful boy who was doing all the wonderful things that little boys do.

However, when Jake was 2, Grace noticed that he seemed different from their friends' children. Jake appeared to have selective hearing. He would respond and pay attention only at certain times. Was this a result of having a history of chronic ear infections? Additionally, at the age of 2, Jake rarely spoke in more than 1- to 2-word utterances, and his language did not expand until he was 3 years old. More perplexing was that he would repeat statements made to him instead of responding to them, as well as mimic what he had heard from the video scene that he insisted on watching constantly. Though Jake would play games with other children, he insisted that they always play them the exact same way. He would seldom initiate or even join in play with other children. These concerns led his parents to seek advice from their pediatrician. They were referred to a speech pathologist, then a speech therapist, and then a clinical psychologist, who was the first person to mention autism. Eventually, they found their way to the office of Dr. B. J. Freeman, a highly regarded diagnostician in the field of autism.

On June 20, 1995, only 4 years and 2 months after Jake was born, he was taken to UCLA for testing. The Wechsler Preschool Primary Scale of Intelligence and the Vineland Adaptive Behavior Scale were administered. Dr. Freeman reported that testing was difficult to administer because Jake would often refuse to complete the tasks. Furthermore, Jake's eye contact was poor throughout the evaluation, and his speech was flat and perseverative in nature. Results of testing revealed that Jake had a Full-Scale IQ of 94, and his Performance IQ (111) was higher than his Verbal IQ (81). The Vineland yielded an adaptive behavior composite score of 3 years, 3 months.

Dr. Freeman explained to Grace and Todd that Jake met the criteria for the diagnosis of autistic disorder. She shared that he appeared to have good skills and outstanding potential. She also shared that one could never be certain about the future. There are so many unpredictable challenges. She recommended that they consider providing Jake intensive intervention based upon Applied Behavior Analysis (ABA).

Grace and Todd were numb. Although they were not shocked to hear the formal diagnosis, since they had already heard the speech therapist say that she suspected it, it was devastating all the same. On the way home, they couldn't even recall what Dr. Freeman had said! How did this happen? Did they do something wrong? Why didn't they get him evaluated sooner? What was the long-term prognosis? What kind of life would he live? Most important, however, was how could they best help him?

Early Intervention Years

The time after a parent is informed that his or her child has autism is excruciating. Besides the obvious, there is tremendous confusion about what to do, especially given all of the contradictory information. It is hard not to feel desperate and therefore willing to participate in any treatment that sounds plausible. Grace and Todd described feeling stranded, alone on a deserted island, with no chance of rescue while at the same time needing to save their child.

The speech therapy that Jake received before the diagnosis had helped him expand his vocabulary and improve his articulation. However, Jake clearly needed more than the 3 hours a week of speech therapy he was receiving. The mother of a classmate at Jake's preschool had given Grace a flyer about a workshop by Autism Partnership. Grace approached one of the authors of this chapter (Dr. Ronald Leaf) at the workshop to see how she could obtain services for her son. Dr. Freeman had suggested that they contact Autism Partnership to see if it could provide services. An appointment was made to get the ball rolling.

The Journey Starts

In the first meeting, I recognized that Jake demonstrated extremely favorable prognostic indicators. He possessed some expressive language and adequate play skills and was socially connected. Moreover, his self-stimulation was highly sophisticated, another positive indicator. I informed Jake's parents that with intensive and quality intervention it was possible that he would have a favorable outcome. However, without intervention, no matter how "high functioning" Jake might be, it was unlikely that he would reach his potential. However, I shared some good news. I felt the progress would be rapid and that intervention would be extremely short term—perhaps no more than a few months.

Grace and Todd expressed their concerns regarding ABA. They had heard that it was a procedure that was ineffective in the long run. They were under the impression that it might produce quick but temporary changes. They also had heard that it was not child friendly and that the majority of the intervention involved drills conducted only while sitting at a table. They did not want Jake to have to sit at a table being drilled for hours and working for candy. They had also heard that it could be punitive, cold, and unnatural. They feared that Jake would become an unhappy child with skills that did not generalize.

I informed Grace and Todd that, unfortunately, this was the reputation and misperception of ABA. There are many misconceptions about ABA, and in some cases these are perpetuated by people in the field who claim to be behavioral specialists. I further explained that good ABA is a positive approach that utilizes natural teaching strategies and that Autism Partnership uses what Dr. Ronald Leaf defined as Contemporary Behavior Therapy. Our motto is "Children cry when the therapists leave, not when they arrive!" Therapy should be fun and inspiring. And when that occurs, children learn, and the learning lasts!

Grace and Todd had renewed hope and agreed that Jake should immediately begin receiving ABA. Although ABA accounted for more than 95% of Jake's intervention, at different times throughout his intervention Jake also received alternative treatments, such as speech therapy, a gluten- and wheat-free diet, and one dose of secretin (a hormone that received a great deal of attention years ago when parents reported improvements following an infusion of secretin; however, research found no differences between children receiving secretin and the control group).

Assessments and observations made at Autism Partnership revealed that Jake had many maladaptive behaviors and skill deficits that needed intervention. Although Jake could be quite verbal, without probing you would not know it. He rarely commented, was not spontaneous, and would give one-word answers to questions. He rarely asked questions and certainly was not conversational. One of the glaring issues was Jake's total lack of interest in children. He was resistant to playing with peers and would not interact socially with children his own age. Additionally, Jake displayed many ritualistic behaviors such as watching the same videotape over and over, playing with the same toy in the same manner, repeating statements made to him, and repeating the lines of his favorite videos and cartoons.

The initial focus of therapy was to reduce Jake's ritualistic play while expanding his language skills. If we were able to increase his appropriate play skills and language, it would facilitate his socialization skills. Obviously, we would be addressing those behaviors that greatly interfered with developing friendships, as well as those that interfered with learning. Therapists would play Jake's favorite games, but gradually they would change the way they played. For example, they varied what color piece they used, who started, and even some of the rules. Continuously, therapists insisted that he use more language, facilitating his spontaneous comments and encouraging him to ask questions. Early success occurred with intervention as Jake started to communicate more appropriately and engaged in fewer ritualistic behaviors.

Though there was some initial success, therapy also revealed additional skills that needed intervention. For example, Jake was extremely competitive and would exhibit tantrum behaviors any time he lost. Jake also became more and more noncompliant with his therapists and his parents, often refusing to participate in therapy or follow requests from his mother. Intervention was implemented to address these issues. For example, Jake received his favorite reinforcers when he graciously lost. He was also reinforced for compliance but would lose his turn when he did not follow instructions. We also began a frustration tolerance program to help address his intolerance for losing, with the eventual goal of teaching him coping skills. His competitiveness was creating social problems, and therefore we felt we needed to address it directly. But the biggest concern was starting to become apparent. Jake was a bundle of emotions. He appeared to be an angry and, sometimes, a very sad little boy. So much for my prediction of a quick intervention!

Years 2 and 3

The next 2 years of therapy had many ups and downs for Jake, his parents, and his therapists. There were wonderful successes, but these were tempered with emerging behavioral challenges. Although his language was exploding and it was extremely clear that he was bright, it also became clear that it was critical that we more directly address his disruptive behaviors. Jake's noncompliance and his attempts to "control the world" were greatly hindering therapy and certainly the development of friendships. Although Jake had outstanding skills, as long as he continued to refuse to listen and withdraw from peers, it really did not matter!

Teaching Jake to become a better listener became a prime objective. To accomplish this goal, a compliance hierarchy was established. Instructions were assigned to one of three categories: those with the highest probability of compliance, those Jake would follow sometimes, and those to which he would rarely respond. If Jake complied with any instruction, he received a great deal of reinforcement. However, if Jake did not follow directions, staff would remain neutral, and he would lose the opportunity to receive reinforcement. This intervention resulted in drastic improvements.

We then expanded the frustration tolerance program. Initially, we taught Jake to recognize when he was feeling angry and when he was happy. We believed that if Jake could become better at identifying his emotions, he would be more able to cope with his frustration. At the same time, we taught him to use guided imagery when he felt mad. Jake learned to think of his favorite cartoon character as soon as he started feeling the least amount of anger. The enjoyment he felt in imagining his favorite character had the effect of reducing his anger. Eventually, the number of situations that triggered frustration was greatly reduced.

We also implemented an extensive play program to reduce Jake's obsession with Star Wars (e.g., perseverating on the topic, insisting on playing only with Star Wars figures). We believed that by expanding his play interests and building new passions, we would reduce his intense interest in Star Wars. We picked interests that other boys his age demonstrated. So soccer and baseball became our focus. We hoped that this would facilitate the development of social relationships. We more directly addressed his social development by increasing his skills in paying attention to his peers, following their lead, and joining in on conversations.

Kindergarten brought on new challenges, new behaviors, and big changes for Jake. The first issue that had to be resolved was whether support staff should go to school with Jake to help ensure success. Although Jake had made tremendous gains and was rapidly approaching becoming indistinguishable from his peers, it was feared that inattention and noncompliance might again creep in and eventually set him apart. Moreover, his fascination with Star Wars could emerge again if we failed to monitor him adequately.

After much deliberation, we determined that it would be in Jake's best interest if staff were present. However, staff members were instructed to be as unobtrusive as possible. There would not be any systematic contingency system, and assistance would be provided only as absolutely necessary. Staff were told that they were to act as if they were "secret agents"; they should become visible only in an emergency. The students and their parents should never be able to detect that they were Jake's shadow; they should be perceived as classroom aides that the school district generously provided for the entire class.

Intervention at school focused mainly on increasing Jake's independence, his ability to attend and learn within a natural group setting, and, of course, his social relationships. More specifically, targeted goals for Jake were to follow group and individual instructions, pay attention to the teacher, stay on task, participate in social interactions, stay in the group, and notice what the other children were doing. Intervention was quite successful. Jake's ability to learn in a group and pay attention to the teacher increased dramatically. He also became quite independent in the classroom. He was able to follow the class rules and schedule and to complete tasks on his own.

Although Jake was having daily triumphs, it was also becoming clear that he was having trouble simply being a child! He was not interacting socially. He would not talk to or even play with his peers. Jake appeared to be uninterested and was unwilling to socialize. It became critical that we develop programs to address these issues, to avoid his being stigmatized as a loner. More important, if we couldn't increase his social interest, we risked serious repercussions that could ultimately affect the quality of his life. Two other issues were emerging: (a) Jake was growing tired of therapy and the demands that were being placed on him, and (b) he exhibited a noticeably sad demeanor in school and at home.

The Elementary School Years

The course became clear. We were no longer concerned about academics and cognitive functioning. The mission was to concentrate all of our efforts on providing Jake with the skills and interests so that he could develop meaningful friendships. Our expectation was that this would successfully address his depression, as well.

We began by exposing Jake to situations that would facilitate his interactions outside school. His parents arranged for play dates at their house. Although it was not always easy to find the right peer and parents who were agreeable, they were persistent in their efforts. This allowed therapists to work on social skills in a more structured setting than was possible in school. In addition, Jake attended a sports camp, which provided him the opportunity to interact with multiple children in a less formal setting. Finally, Jake started to participate in Little League and AYSO, which gave him additional children with whom to interact.

It was critical to develop individualized programs to help Jake learn the prerequisite skills needed to increase social interactions. A "cool–not cool" program was implemented in which Jake had to learn to discriminate between behaviors that were socially acceptable (labeled "cool") and those behaviors that were not socially acceptable ("not cool"). Issues such as sharing, compromising, and not perseverating were targeted. To teach these discriminations, one of his therapists acted out a behavior that was either socially appropriate or a behavior that was socially inappropriate. Jake's job was to tell his therapist if the behavior was "cool" or "not cool." Jake's next responsibility was to demonstrate the behavior in a "cool" manner. Gradually, we began to see slight improvements. Jake was less off-putting in the classroom. However, during recess and lunch and after school, he still remained unapproachable. Nonetheless, we remained encouraged by the slight progress and continued in our efforts.

Week after week, we started seeing Jake becoming more interested in social interaction, both inside and outside the classroom. As Jake became more socially engaged, peer approval became a far more powerful force. His perseverative and highly competitive behaviors started to reduce. Not surprisingly, his peers became more accepting and then interested in him. One peer, Andy, captured his interest. His parents jumped on the opportunity and invited Andy for play dates and outings.

After Jake and Andy became friends, we saw incredible improvements in Jake's social interactions. He was becoming more social during unstructured times (e.g., recess, lunch, and after school), he started to play more with peers, and he was increasing the amount of time that he engaged in play. In addition, the frequency of inappropriate behaviors during social interactions, such as gazing or slight body self-stimulation (e.g., hand movements), decreased dramatically. Jake's exposure to his peers was also expanded, because he now not only participated in baseball and soccer but also started going to his yacht club to sail. Finally, it seemed that we had a handle on his social skills. But the job was far from over. So much for the prediction of a few months or even few years!

It was the goal for Jake's cognitive functioning to continue to stay at grade level despite the tremendous increase in academic difficulty. At the same time, we wanted to decrease the assistance he needed to help him through the school day to avoid his being stigmatized by the additional attention he was receiving. In order for Jake to remain successful in the general education classroom, it was important to make sure that his academic skills were on par with those of his peers. Fortunately, Jake was a very intelligent child who had many strengths and was able to learn new skills and concepts quickly. Although Jake was clearly an intelligent child, he did have some noticeable deficits in comparison to other children in his class. As concepts became more abstract and therefore more difficult for him, he started paying less attention. A majority of the time, Jake would engage in competing behaviors such as gazing, looking down at his desk, or other self-stimulatory behaviors. If Jake did not pay attention to the teacher, clearly he would not be able to learn the material, thereby requiring the need for a behavioral assistant, perhaps for the remainder of his education.

We contemplated many different programs, ranging from subtle to quite intrusive. We had always rejected being intrusive. We simply did not want Jake to be identified as different. But, we felt that he needed extremely comprehensive programs that would require his shadows to provide him constant feedback. We rationalized that his behaviors were already distinguishing him as a student who needed assistance. Also, he had true friends. His friendships were based upon reciprocity and not a sense among his friends that they needed to take care of him or be nice to him. They simply had common interests and wanted to be his friend. So we were slightly less concerned about the repercussions of our being intrusive. We conferred with his parents. They had always been reluctant for him to be identified, but they understood the stakes and gave us their support.

The goal was to eventually decrease Jake's need for behavioral assistance by increasing his attention span when he was presented with difficult material. We also wanted to teach him to be better able to identify when it was important to pay attention and when it was not as important. Most important, we needed to teach Jake to self-monitor his attention. The foundation of the program was that he received tokens when he displayed sustained attention. These tokens were exchanged at home for reinforcers (e.g., watching extra TV, buying baseball cards, playing on the computer).

It became critical for us to transfer assistance provided to Jake from the shadow to his teacher. We desperately wanted to completely fade his shadows by the end of elementary school so that he could attend middle school without any support. A fading program was put into place so that instructional control could transfer from the behavioral assistants to the teacher. The teacher gradually became responsible for providing all instructions as well as feedback. Additionally, if Jake needed assistance, he was to ask the teacher and not his support staff. If for any reason Jake needed help, the behavioral assistants were instructed to give prompts through either a gesture or a nonverbal prompt. The third step of the fading program was for the behavioral assistant to walk around the room and help the other children in the class, forcing Jake to become more independent. We had gone back to secret agent mode. As Jake's success rate increased, the behavioral assistants started to fade out the time that they were in the classroom, gradually increasing the amount of time Jake was in the class without them. Shadows were encouraged to systematically leave the classroom for prolonged periods of time. Eventually, it was planned for them to be "sick" and therefore absent from the classroom.

Once the shadows were away for considerable periods of time, a change was made in the reinforcement system that was being implemented. It was determined that the token system that was being used was too cumbersome for the teacher; it needed to be changed so that both Jake and the teacher would be successful. The token system was switched to a simple self-monitoring system in which Jake was responsible for monitoring his own behavior and the teacher would then agree or disagree with Jake's self-evaluation. The final component of the fading process was the removal of behavioral assistance altogether so that Jake would be in the classroom by himself. In order to make sure that Jake would become successful, behavioral assistants who were unknown to Jake would occasionally go in the classroom pretending to be teacher's aides and would monitor Jake's behavior.

In Jake's last year of elementary school, he was able to participate in the school's annual tradition of sending the fifth graders to a mountain retreat for a week where they were able to learn about nature and the ecology of the mountains. This was something his parents previously could only have dreamed about happening. Additionally, while in the fifth grade, Jake won the school-wide spelling bee. By the end of elementary school, Jake was able to attend the classroom without an aide and was above grade level in all subjects. More important, he continued to have meaningful friendships. It seemed as if everything was going well for Jake, because he was excelling in most areas of his life. However, Jake still continued to exhibit signs of depression. To help

Jake with this concerning area, he started to receive behavioral counseling once a week after school from one of the behavioral supervisors
at Autism Partnership.

The majority of the sessions were devoted to discussing Jake's
recognition of his being slightly different. He realized that it was
harder for him to concentrate than his friends. Also, there were times
that it was hard for him to want to interact. Perhaps his biggest issue
was not wanting to have support, because he was embarrassed and
stressed when people constantly focused on the things that were
"wrong" with him. Jake and his counselor discussed various coping
strategies he could use. They also talked about the typical struggles of
adolescents. But perhaps the most valuable aspect was that Jake was
simply able to talk to someone about his issues. What became clear
was that it was imperative for Jake to understand why he was different
and why he was receiving support. We felt it was essential that he be
informed about his diagnosis and therefore why we were "bugging him."

Naturally, this was not our decision. His parents had not only to
concur but to strongly support such a decision.

Revealing the Diagnosis

Because Jake was originally going to be in intervention for only a short
time, his parents had hoped they would never have to tell him or others beyond the grandparents and a few close friends about his diagnosis. They had started couples counseling in March 1996, when Jake was
almost 5 years old, to deal with the devastating issues that affect a family who has a child with autism—marital stress involving differences in
reactions to the diagnosis and prognosis, the huge demands on time
and the reduced privacy, the wish to keep people from knowing about
the diagnosis and the isolation that that creates—and to just be able to
discuss the emotions elicited by the roller coaster ride involved in
watching one's child go through this enormous struggle. The decision
to tell Jake required that Todd and Grace directly face all of their fears
and sadness about the diagnosis. It was critical that we prepare them
to be able to tell Jake in an open, supportive, and optimistic way.

The parent's therapist, Jake's counselor, and Todd and Grace all
met to strategize about the best way for all to manage this undertaking.
Essentially, a script was developed covering the information that Jake
needed and the points that his parents wanted him to understand

about why this information had been withheld. Everyone brainstormed about possible questions that Jake might have and the best responses to those questions. Having a specific plan for the words to use in the discussion was extremely useful in helping Todd and Grace feel more in control of the situation. Work would begin on preparing Jake for the actual telling and the process that would follow.

In their sessions, Jake's counselor had introduced the importance of being familiar with one's strengths and weaknesses and of understanding that everyone has areas of difficulty. They were coauthoring a story that involved a character who was gifted with various superpowers. The counselor suggested to Jake that maybe they could explore what it would be like if their character also had a learning disability. Famous people who also happened to have disabilities with specific labels were mentioned. Presenting to Jake the reality that facing struggles and figuring out ways to deal with those struggles are a factor in everyone's life was a focus during sessions.

When the agreed-upon time came, Todd and Grace started the conversation with Jake in his bedroom and sailed through the previously dreaded process. After all the anticipation, Jake had few questions and seemed satisfied with the explanation for why he had been receiving all of those annoying therapy sessions for so long. Most notably, he later apologized to his counselor for thinking that the staff had been bugging him for all of those years and what a pain he must have been. It was made clear to Jake that any time he wanted to talk about his autism or had any questions, both his parents and his counselor would be completely available. The hurdle was passed, which was a source of relief for everyone involved, especially his parents.

Moving On

In June 2003, Jake was promoted from elementary school. Standing in front of all the parents, families, and other children, Jake was indistinguishable from his classmates. Shortly afterward, Jake went back to UCLA for another follow-up assessment. This assessment revealed that he had above-average intelligence. But perhaps more exciting was the finding that he was socially adept. He was empathic, sensitive, and socially wise!

Even though this was an exciting time for Jake and his family, it was also a scary time. Jake was now going to be going into middle school, where he would have to deal with several teachers, rather than just one. Middle school also brought more difficult classes, which would require that Jake pay even closer attention. Middle school would prove to be a very exciting and challenging time for Jake.

Any concerns we had were quickly alleviated. Despite being placed in GATE classes and even without supports, he was not only succeeding but was doing "A" work. He was navigating the challenging world of middle school, getting to class on time on a big campus, and being the little fish in the big pond.

Conclusion

In June 2006, Jake walked across the stage and received his promotion certificate from Nobel Middle School. With a big smile on his face, his family taking pictures, and his friends giving him "high fives" on his way off stage, he was so typical that no one could never have guessed all the hard work that had made this moment possible. From the initial assessment at UCLA when Jake was diagnosed as having autism, to the initial meeting at Autism Partnership, to the countless hours of therapy, to the final assessment at UCLA showing that he had reached best outcome, with an IQ of 120, all seemed worthwhile. Now, at the age of 14, Jake will be heading off to a private high school without the support of Autism Partnership and without other than the typical worries about what the future will hold. The future remains bright for Jake— 4 years from now he will be walking across the stage of his high school and preparing to attend any college of his choice—that is, if he can keep from socializing too much!

Nick's Story

Prediagnosis and Noticing Something Different

In the spring of 1997, Grace and Todd were expecting the birth of their third child. Jake was doing well in therapy and had made vast improvements. Grace and Todd could finally feel a little more comfortable that Jake was on the right path. They took great comfort that their daughter, Emily, was doing fine, with no hint of autism. As Grace and Todd eagerly awaited the day of their new arrival, they were guardedly optimistic that they were going to have another healthy child.

Nick, a beautiful baby boy, was born in early April. The joy that the entire family felt was unmatched as they welcomed Nick into their family. Though Nick was reaching many of his developmental milestones within the typical range, his walking was greatly delayed. Moreover, Grace started to believe that Nick was engaging in behaviors similar to those that Jake engaged in prior to his diagnosis.

Was this a case of Grace simply being hypersensitive? How could she not be! Was Nick simply copying some of Jake's behaviors? After all, Nick was clearly different from Jake. He was far more socially engaged. He also was far more interested in playing and communicating.

To Grace, as well as to Jake's behavior therapists, it seemed clear that Nick had a fixation with lights; if left alone, he would ritualistically turn them on and off. But it is not unusual for children to look at lights and fans, and enjoying the control of turning on and off lights is not unusual. Were these really obsessive behaviors, or was everyone just being paranoid? Grace commented that Nick had poor eye contact with both peers and adults, and on occasion he would make abnormal gestures; on the other hand, he was affectionate. Perhaps Grace was being too cautious. Jake's therapists noticed that Nick had language deficits somewhat similar to those that Jake had exhibited. The therapy team appeared to be hypercritical. Providing therapy often makes one suspect that everyone has autistic disorder!

But to be safe and alleviate everyone's panic, Grace and Todd decided to have Nick go to UCLA for formal testing. Even though Nick was only 14 months old, why wait? Once and for all, they wanted to rule out the possibility that there were problems. However, Dr. Freeman and her colleagues experienced the same confusion as everyone else. At times Nick would cry without any apparent provocation, although going through the evaluation process can be upsetting for any 14-month-old. It seemed that his play was somewhat ritualistic, although young children often have their own particular rules around their play. Since Nick was so young, many of the assessment tools proved difficult to implement. An Autism Diagnostic Observation Schedule (ADOS) was administered to determine Nick's functioning level. Though it was clear that Nick had "autistic-like tendencies," Dr. Freeman simply did not feel comfortable making a diagnosis. It was Dr. Freeman's impression that Nick was at risk for autism. It was her recommendation that he could benefit from early intervention with or without a formal diagnosis of autism. After all, what harm could it do to provide stimulation for language, play, and social skills?

Nick's parents wasted no time in arranging for Autism Partnership to immediately start working with their toddler. An immediate hurdle was securing funding for intervention. In California, regional centers often fund such intervention as long as the child meets the eligibility requirements. However, since a diagnosis of autistic disorder could not be made in Nick's case, determining eligibility was far more complicated. It became an issue of whether he had a slight global delay or a language delay—or perhaps everyone was just being overly sensitive. Ultimately, the regional center disagreed with Dr. Freeman, a world-renowned diagnostician, and concluded that Nick did not have any signs of autism. Although they funded physical therapy to target his walking problems, they refused to fund ABA services. Grace and Todd immediately decided they were not going to waste precious time and potentially compromise Nick's life. They decided to pay privately for the services he needed and at some later point attempt to secure funding.

First Year of Therapy

Nick arrived at Autism Partnership for his intake. Our initial observations revealed that Nick was skilled in playing and attending to others. We also noted that Nick would often engage in temper tantrums, perhaps because of his deficits in communication skills or because he was frustrated in his attempts to control his environment.

We recommended that Nick start receiving 15 hours of behavioral intervention a week and noted that gradually we would increase the hours. Initially, we focused on decreasing his disruptive behaviors that interfered with learning. We implemented multiple programs, including a frustration tolerance program. In this program, Nick was systematically exposed to situations that evoked frustration, starting with lower level situations (e.g., being told no, having to stop watching TV, being asked to pick up his toys). We also worked on teaching him how to request what he wanted (e.g., videos, toys, to be left alone). Nick was placed on a rich reinforcement schedule in which he would be reinforced for the absence of behaviors such as aggression, whining, and noncompliance. Reinforcement also occurred when he appropriately coped with frustration and communicated. Our program also placed a great emphasis on expanding his language, such as increasing the length of his utterances and developing spontaneous commenting.

For the first 6 months, Nick flew through programs. It was not unusual for Nick to master targets within a day and entire phases of programs within a week. Therapists were instructed to keep pushing peer interaction, because it was becoming clear that this area was Nick's biggest deficit area. Even though Nick was improving, his aggression and frustration were increasing, despite the programs designed to address these issues.

In March 1999, just 6 months after Nick's initial visit to UCLA, he was reevaluated to assess his progress and to determine whether he met the criteria for autistic disorder. Dr. Freeman administered the Mullens test and found that his visual skills were at 30 months, fine motor skills were at 24 months, receptive language skills were at 23 months, and expressive language skills were at 18 months. Although his development thus was only slightly delayed, the presence of ritualistic play, resistance to change, and limited interest in peers led to his receiving the diagnosis of autistic disorder. Dr. Freeman was pleased with Nick's progress and recommended that he continue to receive behavior therapy to assist him with his language, play skills, and social interactions.

Despite knowing in their hearts that Nick was autistic, Grace and Todd were devastated, nonetheless. Hearing those words made it a reality. They had two boys with autism! Even though they believed both of their sons had a favorable prognosis, it did not eliminate their sadness.

For the next 6 months, our program continued to focus on increasing Nick's compliance by offering reinforcement when he listened and ignoring times when he was noncompliant. Our program also concentrated on teaching Nick prosocial skills such as paying attention and interacting with peers. He was taught how to seek help to avoid his intense frustration when he could not do something. A token economy was put into place in which Nick could receive tokens and, ultimately, reinforcement if he did not display any aggression for a predetermined period of time. Despite Nick's continued aggression, he was responding very well to therapy. He continued to learn rapidly and to use these skills outside therapy. He was able to maintain skills over a long period. Additionally, he now started to seek out his brother and sister when they came home after school. Was it possible that Nick would eventually be indistinguishable from his peers? All of us were keeping our fingers crossed and working as hard as possible to give him his childhood back.

Late in 1999, Nick and Grace made another trip to UCLA for reevaluation. Dr. Freeman was astonished by Nick's growth in a 6-month period. Testing indicated that in 6 months he had made an 11-month increase in his visual skills, an 8-month increase in receptive language, and a whopping 14-month improvement in expressive language. He also improved in all areas except for social skills, as measured on the Vineland Adaptive Behavior Scales.

Second Year

After 1 year of therapy, it was clear that Nick was making substantial improvements. Was it possible that both boys could achieve outcomes similar to those of Catherine Maurice's children (as described in her book *Let Me Hear Your Voice*)? Todd and Grace realized that it might be premature to dream that far ahead, but their optimism was essential to keep them in this war.

The 2nd year's mission was to make therapy as natural as possible. We wanted to get Nick into preschool as quickly as possible and to have him participate in typical activities for 3-year-olds. Therefore, it was essential for his skills to continue to generalize. Instructions had to be natural, reinforcement had to closely approximate what he would encounter in preschool or on play dates, and he had to become less dependent on adults for help. Also of paramount importance, his aggression had to be eliminated!

A time-in program was implemented in order to address Nick's aggression. Nick wore a watch that symbolized that he was able to access reinforcement on a frequent basis. If he displayed any form of aggression or whining, then the watch was immediately removed and he lost access to all reinforcement. In order to earn the right to have the watch back, he had to remain calm and follow instructions for 15 minutes. This program proved to be highly successful, and it seemed that the aggression battle might have finally been won.

By eliminating Nick's aggression, we were better able to focus on his social skills. He was placed in the social skills group program at Autism Partnership. This was an afterschool program that included typically developing peers. The purpose of the program was to teach children with autism how to appropriately interact with peers. Skills such as initiating, sharing, and compromising were targeted. This program uses typically developing peers and trained staff who can teach in a group format. Such a program provided Nick with a more natural manner to learn social skills, in addition to providing him access to many same-age peers.

Nick was making such good progress that his mom made an unusual request. She wanted to see what would happen if we stopped therapy for 2 months. Not only did she feel she and Nick needed a break, but she wanted him to have a normal life. She wanted him to stop missing social opportunities. After all, how could he develop friendships if he could not go to his friends' houses because of therapy? She wanted to be able to go to the park with him and just be his mom. Her arguments were compelling. He was doing so well, and her point about having more normal interactions with children was hard to argue with. So we thought it would be a good test. It was a win-win arrangement. If he continued to improve without intervention, that would be fabulous. If he regressed, then we would know the course we had to take.

After a 2-month break from therapy, Nick began to regress. He was becoming less expressive and far less social. More problematic was the return of aggression, noncompliance, and tantrums. It was clear that Nick was not ready for termination. Although he had made amazing progress, it was also clear that we had a lot of work to do. With renewed vigor, we once again began providing 35 hours of intervention weekly. Nick immediately responded. It was as if he had not missed a day. His disruptive behaviors rapidly decreased, while his language and social skills returned.

At the end of the year, when Grace was asked to describe Nick in an assessment, she stated, "For a child who has had about half of his life in therapy, Nick is an inspiration to those who know him. Although he has had his moments, he is a bright, shining, and an adorable young guy. At age three he has accomplished a lot."

Third Year

The third year of therapy consisted of fine-tuning Nick's communication skills and teaching him more advanced social skills. Nick was certainly interested in his peers and even enjoyed play dates. But he lacked some important skills that could help him develop more and deeper friendships. The language curriculum we implemented consisted of expanding his language so that he would be more descriptive in his sentence use, teaching him the correct use of pronouns, and having him ask questions to seek information from his peers. In conjunction with asking questions, Nick was taught how to make advanced inferences (e.g., if Billy likes Batman, Superman, and Spiderman, he would probably rather play with the "X-Men" toys than play baseball) so that he would be able to play games that his friends wanted to play. Additional targeted areas for development were skills such as sportsmanship, conflict resolution, abstract reasoning, appropriately joining a group, and relaxation—all of which were eventually acquired.

The most important aspect of therapy was to facilitate Nick's success in preschool. We suspected that this would be no easy task. The school's philosophy was to provide very little structure and to have children learn from exposure. Moreover, any problems between the children were to be worked out between themselves. While this philosophy may be feasible with most children, we did not suspect that it would work for Nick. To complicate matters, the school administrators were not eager to have staff shadow Nick. Reluctantly, they allowed us to observe occasionally and intervene only if absolutely necessary.

Our observations in the preschool setting revealed that Nick regularly played with a variety of children and was willing to play a variety of games. There were times, however, when he was very bossy to his friends, ordering them around or setting up his own rules for games. Although Nick was very conversational with his friends and would join in on a variety of topics, he usually talked about Star Wars and Harry Potter. Compliance was not a huge issue for Nick, although he would often attempt to pressure his peers to complete tasks for him. During circle time, Nick's attention span was equal to that of any of his peers. His teachers claimed that Nick was indistinguishable from his peers. Had he reached best outcome?

Fourth and Fifth Year

Nick entered public school. He was enrolled in a general education kindergarten classroom. The school allowed us to provide support staff to help in the transition. There was no dictated timetable of when they would be faded. Nick's performance would dictate the plan.

In August 2003, Nick went back to UCLA for follow-up testing. The WISC IV test revealed that Nick had a Full-Scale IQ of 119, which put him in the 88th percentile. His global functioning score improved by 40 points to a score of 90, revealing that his quality of life had increased substantially since he started receiving therapy. Though Dr. Freeman concluded that he still presented as a child with autistic disorder, he had made vast improvements. Although he did not meet the criteria of "best outcome," since he still presented as autistic, it would be hard for anyone but the most trained professional to identify the remaining challenges.

The next 2 years of intervention consisted of increasing Nick's flexibility. Nick was very inflexible in playing games with his friends or when he was talking to his friends. For Nick, conversations had to flow a certain way, and games needed to be played how they were intended to be played, leaving no room for imagination. These two behaviors were setting him apart from his peers. Our therapists began to play games by not following the rules of the game. If he was not oppositional to such changes, he would receive reinforcement. Within a few months, although he still preferred to be rule oriented, Nick became much more flexible with his play. Our therapy also concentrated on teaching Nick how to lose graciously, how to be more cooperative, and how to expand his friendships from one special friend to multiple peers.

Within short order Nick had multiple friends that he hung out with at school and home. Like his brother, Jake, he started playing Little League baseball and AYSO soccer and was quite a good athlete. During the summer, he attended the local sports camp, which he loved and which also helped him expand his friendships to peers outside his school. He was actually one of the most popular children in school. Academically, he was one of the top students in the class, excelling in all subjects. Although he could be easily distracted, he could also be redirected quite easily. It was time to fade and then eliminate his support services.

A fading plan was put in place so that by February of first grade Nick would no longer have support staff with him at school. Moreover, he would no longer be receiving direct behavioral intervention at home. The plan consisted of initially having shadow support at school with him 100% of the time. It was hoped that this level would be reduced to 60% by the end of kindergarten. By November of first grade, support staff were at school to support him only 40% of the time, with elimination by February. Throughout this period, our staff were to provide assistance only if absolutely necessary. Indeed, in February, there was no need for support staff. Nick was observed at random times during school by Autism Partnership staff who were unknown to him. Though he received no direct services, his program supervisor still consulted with his teacher in order to monitor his behaviors and performance and to assist the teacher in any way necessary.

The Final 2 Years

Nick entered second grade without shadow support, no in-home behavior therapy, and very little consultative services. Autism Partnership staff would occasionally observe Nick without his knowledge. Our staff reported that he continued to be popular and stay well above grade level in his subjects, and he was successfully able to self-monitor his behaviors. It was looking as if it would not be long until Nick was no longer a client of Autism Partnership.

However, midway through Nick's second-grade year, his teacher began to notice a resurfacing of negative behaviors. Nick had begun being bossy again, he was slipping in certain academic areas, and he was engaging in ritualistic and inappropriate behaviors. Instead of playing with the group of friends that he usually did, he was hanging around one child in particular and was perseverating on Pokémon.

At the end of the school year, Nick did not receive an invitation to a friend's birthday party. This hit Nick hard. Nick's program supervisor explained to him that if he did not hang around *all* of his friends, his invitations would be limited. He was offered a chance to come back to the social skills group twice a month to work on these issues. Nick decided to take this opportunity and rejoined the social skills group. It was as if Nick needed a wakeup call and just a little bit of structure. His behaviors immediately improved. Nick was back, popular and excelling. He and his parents decided he should continue participating in the social club. They felt it could not hurt. He enjoyed attending, was continuing to learn valuable skills, and was giving back to the "community." He served as a "typical" peer.

Conclusion

Though Nick is still receiving some form of behavioral intervention, his treatment team, Dr. Freeman, and, most important, his parents consider that he has achieved best-outcome status. He is testing at superior levels, and he is totally indistinguishable from his peers at school. Most important, he is an extremely happy little boy who is now able to live the life that his parents dreamed about the day he was born. The road has not been easy. If not for his parents' unrelenting efforts, his treatment team's dedication, and, most important, Nick's determination, Nick would probably not be where he is today.

9

Why Artie Can't Learn!

A teacher presents the following lesson in a hypothetical preschool classroom in everyday Americana:

Teacher: Today we are going to learn about prepositions. I have a large box in the middle of the room. Does everyone see the box? We will use that box. Listen carefully. When I call your name, stand up and see if you can follow my direction. I want Sarah to stand up. [Sarah stands up.] Good, Sarah, I want you to stand in front of the box. Show us where "in front of" the box is.

Sarah: [Demonstrates correct behavior by getting in front of the box. Artie is looking at a discolored spot on the drop ceiling.]

Teacher: Good, Sarah. You stood in front of the box. You did not stand behind the box. Class, did Sarah stand on the box?

Most of class: No.

Teacher: Where did Sarah stand?

Kid raising hand: She stood in front of the box.

Teacher: Let's try another one. Bobby, stand up. [Bobby complies and stands up.] Good, Bobby, I want you to stand behind the box. Show us where to stand so that you are "behind" the box [vocal emphasis on "behind"].

Bobby: [Walks to the box and stands behind it.]

Teacher: Very good, Bobby. You stood behind the box. You did not stand in front of the box. Class, did Bobby stand inside the box?

Most of class: No.

Teacher: Where did Bobby stand?

Kid raising hand: He stood behind the box.

Teacher: [Stops lesson, seeing Artie is still looking at the ceiling and has not paid attention during this entire time.] Artie, you need to pay attention. How can you learn where "in front of" is if you don't watch! [Artie still does not attend.]

Teacher: [Moves closer to Artie.] OK. Artie, get behind the box.

Artie: [Gets up and piles inside the box.]

Teacher: Now see, Artie, if you were listening, you would have gotten behind the box, instead of inside the box. Now pay attention so you can learn the difference between "inside," "in front of," and "behind."

In reviewing this scenario, ask yourself which students profited from this lesson.

- Did Sarah learn?
- Did Bobby learn?
- Did Artie learn?
- Why did Artie not learn?

Perhaps you have seen children like Artie in preschool classes, children who do not attend while a lesson is being presented. Attending skills in the early grade levels are critical to academic success. Listening to the teacher and observing the teacher and/or other students as they demonstrate a skill, such as placing an object in a box rather than outside the box, is critical to skill acquisition in preschool. One-to-one direct teaching, that is, individual prompting requiring the child's attention, is not usually provided. Rather, instruction is geared toward the entire group via the oral presentation of a lesson. In the scenario presented, it was hoped that the children who watched their classmates get up and place themselves in a position relative to the box would learn the relational concept involved in prepositions. The ability to acquire skills by observing others has been termed "observational learning." Much of what young children learn comes through observation. If a child does not attend in the first place, it is hard for him or her to learn observationally.

Artie's ability to profit from this form of instruction is very limited. He does not attend to the verbal presentation by the teacher. He does not observe his classmates performing the requested behavior. Subsequently, he will probably be unable to imitate those actions when asked. If his ability to observe and imitate the behavior performed by another child or a teacher does not improve, will he be any further along in his acquisition of prepositional relations?

Looks Good but Smells Bad!

While traditional forms of teaching and instruction for preschool children may look great, their efficacy with young children with autism is minimal at best. Is it wise to deploy an instructional approach whose prerequisite for success is good attending skills on the part of the child? Does that make sense for children like Artie, whose attending skills are minimal to nil? Here is a hypothetical example of looking good but smelling bad.

The Itsy-Bitsy Spider

It is the start of the class time as all the children arrive in their special education preschool classroom. The five students in the class have autism, with severe adaptive and cognitive deficits. Only one of them says words, but not in any useful or functional sense (she repeats "mama" every so often). The class is heavily staffed, with a credentialed teacher and two instructional aides.

It is the beginning of the day, and that means "the morning circle," a staple in everyday preschool programs for language-capable children. Such a format in a regular preschool class with language-capable children conjures up an image of children learning through doing and saying. But this is a special education class with language-deficient children. The teacher walks over to the CD player, pushes in the play button, while all five children are seated in a semicircle around the teacher's chair at the front of the carpet area. The instructional aides, whose job is to help keep the children in their seat (no small feat), are seated behind the children. The music comes on:

The itsy-bitsy spider went up the water spout...

Any observer to this class sees the following. Of the five students in the class, four at any one time are engaged in some other distracting activity such as hand weaving, turning around, tantrumming, or getting out of their seat. All the children seem oblivious to the concept that this is a learning activity and continue to not attend as the music plays on. One student makes eye contact with the teacher for a while. But within a second he gets up and starts jumping around, at which time he is directed by the nearest adult to sit back down.

The aides are in rhythm and sing their hearts out, following the lead of the teacher. But what also is apparent is the lack of vocal responding from the five students. Of course, one might expect this given that four of them have no capability to produce intelligible words. Even the child who does speak on occasion does not join in but rather seems interested in the knot in her shoelaces. Are the children supposed to be singing? One could make a convincing argument that the production of words via sing-song is a great way to enhance a young child's sophistication in language. But there is a caveat: You have to be able to produce words and actively engage in the activity to learn.

A naive conception among many personnel who work with children with severe disabilities is that repeated practice using this group approach will eventually work. They believe that children like Artie just take longer to learn. Hence, they do these group activities month after month, year after year. When asked, these people proclaim, "He will get it eventually; it just takes more time and patience." Four years later, Artie (now age 8) still does not sing the first five words of "The Itsy-bitsy Spider." What did they mean by getting it eventually?

Why Is Group Daily Practice Not the Answer for Artie?

An interesting series of experiments sheds light on this learning enigma of children with autism. In a nationally renowned multiyear project in the 1960s that investigated effective treatments for autism, Lovaas and his colleagues (1971) addressed this issue. His team attempted to discern why children with autism often took a long time to acquire a target skill, even when being directly taught by an experienced behavior therapist (Lovaas, Koegel, & Schreibman, 1979). These researchers conducted an experiment in two phases. In the first phase, each child was taught to press a bar when one target stimulus (called a discriminative stimulus) was presented and not to press the bar in its absence. The discriminative stimulus was made up of three elements (called a compound stimulus): (a) a moderately bright visual light (red floodlight), (b) an auditory stimulus (white-noise sound), and (c) a tactile event (pressure cuff on child's leg). Here is what this phase of the study looked like. Imagine that the child is in the experimental room with the therapist. The child is taught to press a bar when all three of these elements are presented simultaneously. The act of pressing the bar when all three elements are presented results in food reinforcement. No food reinforcement is presented for bar pressing in the absence of this presentation. The research study encompassed training on this simple discrimination to three groups of children: (a) "normal" children, (b) children with mental retardation, and (c) autistic children.

Children in all three of the groups acquired this discrimination. All children pressed the bar when all three elements were presented simultaneously and did not press the bar in their absence. A reasonable person would assume that all these children had come to equate any of the elements as the basis for responding. In other words, the child attended to all three elements (light, white noise, and pressure on leg) equally, and his or her response was under the control of any and all of these elements.

The second phase of the study tested that notion. In this phase, each element was presented in isolation to see whether its presence would evoke the bar press (this was called single-cue testing). The single-cue test involved 70 presentations of one of the elements (probably divided equally) to each child. For each presentation, the experimenter noted whether the child pressed the bar when a given element was presented. For example, in this phase, the white noise would come on and then end. Sometime later, the light would come on and then be terminated. The number of times the child pressed the bar in the presence of each element (light, white noise, and pressure cuff on the leg) was tabulated.

The results were astounding. The nonhandicapped children (called "normal" in the study) responded to each of the elements equally. In other words, whether the light, white noise, or pressure to the leg was presented singly, the child pressed the bar. In contrast, the children with autism pressed the bar primarily to just one of the elements; three of these children responded to the auditory stimulus, while two would press the bar only when presented with the red floodlight. None of the children with autism responded to the pressure cuff. This "restricted focus" distinguished these children from their nonhandicapped same-aged peers.[14] Had the autistic children attended to only one of the elements to the exclusion of the other two during Phase I training? It seemed so! Similar results regarding restricted focus were found in other studies that examined other aspects of compound stimuli (Lovaas et al., 1979; Koegel & Wilhelm, 1973). The inability of children with autism to attend to multiple elements (or features) of a compound

---

14 This quality is termed stimulus overselectivity in the research study.

stimulus is certainly demonstrated in these series of studies. But what does it mean?

What Are the Implications for Teaching Children With Autism?

In one word, the implications are profound! First, to get the attention of a child with autism is not an easy task. It requires instructional procedures that target his or her initial attention with task presentation. Hence, even small-group teaching strategies do not ensure that, since it is hard to get initial and sustained attention when working with several children at once. If the child is not attending to your instructional presentation, bet dollars to dimes that she is not going to learn the task, irrespective of how much practice she is given every day. However, even if you get attention to an instructional command in one-to-one training, the child may still not learn the skill. If she attends to an irrelevant piece of the instruction, even repeated practice will be futile in helping her acquire the skill. An example best illustrates this.

Let us say you are trying to teach a child with autism to discriminate a request for a coat from a request to get shoes. You will attempt to teach the child to respond differentially to the two different commands, "Pick up the coat" and "Pick up the shoes," as both the coat and the shoes are lying on the bed. Although this seems a fairly simple skill to acquire, these commands are made up of multiple elements. In addition to nonverbal actions that may or may not accompany these commands, there are four words (in English) for each command.

Given these two commands, what element (or feature) tells one what behavior is being requested? In other words, what is the most critical element to focus on in order to get this right? The answer is the last word of each command: "coat" and "shoes." Remember that while one may believe the child is attending to all the elements of these commands, if the child is autistic, he is probably attending to one element within the compound stimulus. If he focuses on the last word uttered and discerns the different syllables involved in each ("coat" vs. "shoes"), he will learn this task.

But suppose the child focuses on the word "pick." Unfortunately for this child, "pick" is inherent in both commands. Therefore, unless he attends to a different element, he will only be able to guess which article of clothing to pick up. Correcting his mistake will prove fruitless. He will continue to not learn the task, despite day after day of practice on that skill. His attending to only one element in this compound stimulus will keep him from mastering this simple discrimination. In my clinical work with children with autism, I have found that it is often the case that they ignore all the different unique phonemes of the English language that make up words.

This results in the illusion of learning when children with autism respond correctly to a designated task. Let me illustrate with the teaching example just presented. Suppose the tone or voice volume that the trainer or parent uses for the command "Pick up the shoes" is markedly louder than the tone used for the command "Pick up the coat." The child may look like she has learned the difference between the two commands, but again it is just an illusion. When she hears a loud voice volume, she picks up the shoes. When she hears the teacher present a command in a softer voice, she picks up the coat. She makes her decision on what to pick up by listening intently to the voice volume, not the syllables of the last word.

It is now obvious what is wrong with this manner of learning. When other people do not use the same differential voice volume for each of these two commands, the child appears to have not learned at all. Again, what she actually learned is that the louder voice volume means that she should pick up the shoes, while the softer volume means that she should pick up the coat.

Let's look at another example and examine the ramifications of restricted focus. The illustration presents two white cards that a teacher might use to teach a child to learn to read the printed numbers 1 and 2. How does any child learn the difference, saying "one" when presented with the card having the number 1 on it and "two" for the other card? By attending to the difference between the form of the number 1 and that for the number 2, right? He might learn that with a vertical line he says "1" when asked what number it is. In contrast, the number with the curve is the element he uses to respond differently; that is, he says "2." Attending to those single elements with the numbers 1 and 2 will be fine as long as the lesson does not proceed to other numbers.

Discrimination task.

When the instructional program proceeds to other numbers that share a similarity with those elements (e.g., "4" with the number 1 and "3" with the number 2), life will become more difficult. What might he say when asked what the number "3" is? You guessed it. He might say "2." If he is to acquire more sophistication with reading numbers, he will have to make his selection on the basis of critical differences in the other elements of these two numbers.

Let's complicate this example even further. Suppose this child does not attend to the form of the numbers. He ignores those elements. Rather, he just sees two rectangle-shaped cards with something printed on them. Looking at the shape of the cards that have the printed number will be no help in responding correctly. Over time, he demonstrates differential responding to these two numbers. Can we assume that he has learned these two numbers? Such responding may just be an illusion of skill acquisition. Suppose, as the school year wears on, the card with the number "1" gets ripped at the corner (whereas the card with the number 2 is not ripped at the corner). He begins to use that difference as a basis for answering "1" when presented that card and "2," when he is presented the non ripped card. Of course, a new set of cards with these two numbers makes his skill "go away." You can see that his "restricted focus" on a single, unfortunately irrelevant element in this task will be to his detriment in acquiring the skill of reading numbers.

What do these examples demonstrate? As long as the child with autism continues to focus on one (possibly irrelevant or redundant) element within any given compound stimulus, she will never learn the concept you are trying to teach. You could give weeks, months, or years of teaching to a target skill on and get nowhere. *With children with autism, it matters how you teach, not just that you teach. All teaching strategies are not created equal!*[15] The cases presented in this book illustrate how much progress can be made when the instructional method takes this phenomenon into account.

---

15 Many cases of successful ABA treatment identify this learning deficiency and use a strategy that gets the child to acquire skill in attending to multiple elements within a compound stimulus by progressively altering the complexity and sophistication of the discrimination tasks being taught.

Appendix A
Why Is Joint Attention Important?

Joint attention is one of the earliest emerging social behaviors in typically developing children. Deficits in joint attention are apparent even before the first spoken word in infants. What makes joint attention so important is its uniqueness to autism. Children with autism use gestures to make their requests known but do not use those same gestures to share experiences in their world. Because deficits in joint attention are present in the majority of children with autism, it is now thought to be one of the earliest and most reliable indicators of this disorder. The earliest forms of joint attention are nonverbal, such as shifting gaze between an object or event in the environment and a familiar person. As in the butterfly example, described in chapter 3, the purpose of these gaze shifts is to share the experience with another person. These behaviors are followed closely by showing toys to others by holding the toy out with an extended hand. Infants then begin to follow others' attention by looking where others gaze or point. As development progresses, children exhibit more advanced levels of joint attention by combining gaze shifts with talking about what they see and using pointing gestures to make sure the familiar adult is sharing the same experience.

Joint attention can be defined in terms of the social nature of its consequence. The goal in joint attention is purely to share attention or interests. Eye contact and gestures in this case are exhibited by the two participants as a means for engaging in sharing an experience. In contrast, a child can use eye contact and gestures to request, for example, a cookie on the shelf. It is important to differentiate the declarative nature of joint attention skills from instrumental social communicative behavior such as nonverbal requesting. The former behavior is the target of concern.

Summary of Joint Attention Curriculum Sequence

Responding to Joint Attention Curriculum

- Maintain sustained eye contact with partner
- Follow a contact point (pictures in a book)
- Follow distal point (toys around the room)
- Follow eye gaze (toys around the room)
- Follow eye gaze within a conversation

Initiating Joint Attention Curriculum

- Request preferred item, using coordinated eye gaze shifts
- Solicit attention to request
- Maintain joint attention during reading (point, gaze shift, comment)
- Show during play (show, gaze shift, comment)
- Solicit attention to show off
- Track conversational speakers (follow speaker and answer questions)
- Initiate contextually related conversation (coordinated eye gaze between referent and adult)

Appendix B
Parent Manual for the *Get Me Game*[16]

ENNIO CIPANI, PhD[17]

Goal: To develop an initial level of compliance to your instructions and commands involving getting requested items, putting items in a specified place and stopping an activity. For children with autism and severe disabilities, this game is well suited to developing the rudiments of instruction-following behavior to simple requests and commands.

The objectives of the *Get Me Game* are:

1. Increase the child's compliance to your instructions involving "get," "put", and "stop."

2. Increase the child's attending and subsequent compliance skills to multiple sequential instructions, that is, lengthier compliance conditions.

Materials Needed: Common items, for example, wearing apparel, silverware, toys, and so on.

Setting/Context: Can be conducted in the living room area in the home, with a table that is easily accessible to the child. Ensure motivation by invoking Grandma's Rule (see explanation below).

Insuring Child Motivation to Play the Game—Grandma's Rule: In order to accrue benefits to compliance in everyday situations, it is

---

16 For technical assistance in implementing the *Get Me Game*, you can contact a Board Certified Behavior Analyst (BCBA) at www.bacb.com. For more serious mental health issues, contact your pediatrician or a professional mental health provider.

17 This manual is adapted from the Behavior Games Home Program with permission.

imperative that you play the *Get Me Game* regularly, meaning daily. You cannot hope to achieve a significant change in your child's compliance if the *Game* is played sporadically. For children with autism, it is necessary for the *Game* to be played daily, perhaps once in the morning and once in the later part of the day.

It is therefore essential that a highly preferred activity follow the successful playing of the game. This specialized contingency is termed Grandma's Rule. The easiest method of doing this is to play the *Game* before a highly preferred daily routine activity. For example, you might schedule the *Get Me Game* before the child's favorite cartoons in the afternoon. The relationship between playing the *Get Me Game* and being allowed to watch afternoon cartoons is the following: If your child does not play the game, refuses to play the *Game*, or quits before the end, no cartoons (i.e., until the game is played). If your child is successful in completing the requirements of the game before the start time of the cartoons, then your child is permitted to watch them. Be sure to allow sufficient time for your child to finish playing the game before cartoon time. If he or she initially refuses and then decides to eventually engage in the game and complete the requirements, he or she can watch whatever is left of the cartoons.

Format of the Game—Get Commands: Set the game up by placing a few common items (e.g., toothbrush, pencil, book, and comb) on a table surface within view. If the child currently has no receptive ability with the items, you will use a point gesture concurrent with the command to indicate to your child the item you desire.[18] A chair is placed several feet away from the table. Your child sits down on the chair. Tell your child that the goal of the game is to earn a designated number of pennies by getting the item requested.

Proceed as follows:

1. Get in close proximity to the child (especially for the first few sessions of playing the game).

2. Get the child's attention by calling his/her name and/or some other signal (e.g., "Look at me, Ready to play?") and don't issue a get command until direct eye contact is obtained.

---

18 If this does not work, put only one item out to "get" for you, the goal at this point is to develop instructional control.

3. Praise the child for attending initially (and intermittently throughout game).

4. Give a short concise command, for example, "Get me the ____." Specify which item the child is to obtain. For children who do not have receptive ability, you would point or gesture the specific item.

5. If your child gets the item requested, praise him/her and drop a penny in the jar.

6. If an error occurs or a failure to comply occurs, initiate the error correction procedure (see explanation below).

7. Play the game until the child has obtained the preset number of pennies.

Each time the child complies correctly with the command, he or she is given a penny. This immediate consequence of performing the requested behavior provides an incentive for the child to continue his or her compliance to "get" commands. It also allows you to designate the completion criterion for the game. A specified number of pennies, earned through compliance to "Get" commands, are required for successful completion of the game. Once this amount has been achieved, the child not only completes the game successfully but also accesses a high-preferred activity (see Grandma's Rule above) possibly along with a bonus prize (especially in the beginning).

For example, you may want to use 6 pennies as the requirement to complete the *Get Me Game*. The child successfully completes the *Game* when he or she has earned 6 pennies. This criterion for completion focuses on the actual number of times the child has complied with a request.

The actual number you require to complete the game should take into account your child's current ability to comply. For some children, 6 pennies might be a reasonable start point. For others, 8 might make the best sense. For some children with autism who might be younger or more impulsive, 2 pennies might be established as the initial requirement.

In the case of children who may not have counting skills, you might want to use a different system. Start with two jars (of different colors), one that contains the designated number of pennies needed to finish and one that is empty. With each correct compliant act, move one penny to the previously empty jar. When all the pennies have been moved, the child has completed the requirements of the *Get Me Game*. This may make it easier for the child to discern how much compliant behavior is required for successful completion.

The initial length of time you play the *Get Me Game* with your child may only be a few minutes. For example, if the completion criterion were for the child to earn 5 pennies, it would not take long. Start with a completion requirement that the child will most likely succeed at. However, it is of primary importance that the game is played until the child earns the necessary pennies before accessing the Grandma's Rule activity. This teaches the child to persist until the task is completed.

Be happy with small successes in the beginning. Some children may be able to start playing the *Game* with a criterion of earning ten pennies, some cannot start that high. Try to ensure that the completion requirement is not overwhelming in the beginning. It is more important to be successful. This game can develop greater levels of sustained compliance once it gets off the ground. However, do not change the completion requirement in the middle of the *Game*! This teaches the child that unmotivated performance on his part changes your behavior. Make the decision to change the requirement in the subsequent games. Therefore, start with a smaller requirement, and build upwards.

Once the child has succeeded reliably with the initial requirement, you can progressively increase the number of pennies needed to complete the game. When the child is earning a sufficient number of pennies (e.g., 15 pennies), you can switch to a time requirement. Switching to a time requirement for completion approximates instructional conditions in a classroom. For example, a child starts with 5 minutes as the completion requirement (after being successful on the penny system). This child must play the *Game* for 5 minutes without interruption in order to earn the high-preferred activity. After the child has been successful for six out of eight days with 5 minutes as the criterion, the parent increases the length of time to 6 minutes. This process of progressively increasing (slightly) the length of the *Get Me Game* is a function of the child's success with the prior time requirement. Once this value becomes lengthy (e.g., 10 minutes), other behavior games (Memory Game, Good Listening Game) can be included in these sessions.

Error Correction Procedures: If an error occurs, that is, the child gets the wrong item or wanders from the area (e.g., gets sidetracked), utilize the following error correction procedure *immediately:*

1. Take the wrong item and place it back on the table, and move the child back to the starting position (no need to explain).
2. Repeat the previous instruction, for example, "Get the pencil!"
3. Guide (either by shadowing or moving with him/her) the child to select the correct item and bring it back.
4. Confirm the correct selection, for example, "Yes, you got the pencil!" and reward with praise and a penny.
5. Present the next command.

The error correction procedure for wandering responses is the same as above, with the addition of a short wait period after Step 1. This provides a brief time out for such a behavior.

Getting Expressive Compliance[19]: Once the child has brought the requested item, ask, "What do you have in your hand?" If needed, prompt the desired response. Depending on the age and expressive language level of the child, you can require either a single-word response, for example, "shoe" or a more sophisticated complete response, for example, "I have a shoe in my hand." The child earns the penny after complying with the command to get the requested item and verbally responding correctly to the question asked.

Error Correction Procedures for Expressive Compliance: If an error occurs, that is, the child identifies the item incorrectly or doesn't respond at all; use the following error correction procedure:

1. Repeat the previous instruction, for example, "What do you have in your hand?"
2. Present the answer for the child to imitate, for example, "I have a shoe in my hand." The child should respond to this form of help before you move to Step 3 below.

---

19 Verbal compliance to be used only if child has expressively labeling skills via vocal or sign language; you may need to contact a BCBA for advice on how to implement this section with your particular child.

3. When the child imitates the answer correctly, confirm the correct response, for example, "Yes, you have a shoe in your hand!" and reward with praise and a penny.

4. Repeat the request again to see if the child responds correctly, that is, "What do you have in your hand?" If he or she responds without any help (e.g., "I have a shoe"), move to another instruction in the next trial. If not, use the error correction procedure delineated above two to three times before moving to another instruction.

Instructional Sequence for the *Get Me Game*: The initial instructional plan might start with a few simple get commands (depends on the age of the child). These commands should be ones in which the child already knows the item, to facilitate the probability of success. Realize that this compliance game is intended to build compliance and attending skills initially.

Once the child learns the game and begins to respond correctly, more difficult items (including pictures) can be used. When the child has acquired compliant behaviors, the focus of the game can shift to more complex instructions. Using questions that require a greater level of processing from the child allows you to begin to develop the child's ability to concentrate, without becoming distracted and engaging in interfering behaviors. Again, the age of the child and developmental level needs to be taken into account.

The following requests, which develop a greater ability to concentrate and process information, can be used in place of simply asking for the item:

• Function questions: "Go get the item we write with," "Go get the item that we cut paper with."

• Classification questions: "Go get the item that belongs in the class of silverware." "Go get the items that are not silverware."

• Position: "Get the item that is in front of the picture of the dog." "Get the fork that is second from the left."

If you see that your child is unfamiliar with the basic concept, you may need to teach the child by prompting the correct or desired response initially, that is, show him or her the right answer. Use the same error correction procedure as delineated previously. If you need help with how to teach new forms of language using the *Get Me Game*, you can contact a BCBA.

Extending the *Get Me Game*: Once the *Get Me Game* develops basic compliance to simple get requests, it can be expanded to simulate real-life conditions and everyday commands in the home environment. The following areas might be considered for the *Get Me Game*.

- Ask the child to get more than one item per command: "Get the red crayon and the blue paper."

- Play the *Get Me Game* with items placed in another room. The format remains the same except the child gets the item requested (where it is normally kept) and brings it back to you. This should be played only after compliance to the *Get Me Game* with items obtained in the same room is reliably occurring.

- Initiate "put" command training. Ask the child to put items in a designated place (from the table or training area). For example, "Put this toothbrush in the bathroom cabinet," or "Put these shoes in mom's closet."

- Initiate "stop" training. Interrupt the child's compliance with another command, for example, "Wait a minute. I want you to put the baseball cards in the drawer first." Obviously, this training should be done after the child has reached mastery on "get" and "put" commands. "Stop" training further develops instructional control by extending compliance to situations where the child needs to halt or desist from an activity. Once the child is able to comply with an instruction following an interruption, "stop" training can be generalized to other situations. One area of application is when the child has to stop a preferred activity, for a short period of time. Shortly after the child is engaged in a more preferable activity, ask the child to stop and comply with another short request. For example, "Charles, can you stop playing ball for a minute and put this paper in the trash." Reinforce such compliance by having a point system for compliance across everyday situations.

Appendix C
Resources

The following books provide general information about autism:

Autism (developmental clinical psychology and psychiatry) by Laura Ellen Schreibman

Autism spectrum disorders: The complete guide to understanding autism, Asperger's syndrome, pervasive developmental disorder, and other ASDs authored by Chantal Sicile-Kira

Thinking in pictures (expanded, tie-in edition): My life with autism (Vintage) authored by Temple Grandin

The way I see it: A personal look at autism and Asperger's by Temple Grandin

Autism's false prophets: Bad science, risky medicine, and the search for a cure authored by Paul A. Offit

Growing up on the spectrum: A guide to life, love, and learning for teens and young adults with autism and Asperger's by Lynn Kern Koegel and Claire LaZebnik

A practical guide to autism: What every parent, family member, and teacher needs to know by Fred R. Volkmar and Lisa A. Wiesner

Assessment of autism spectrum disorders authored by Sam Goldstein, Jack A. Naglieri, and Sally Ozonoff

The everyday advocate: Standing up for your autistic child by Areva Martin

Books Based on ABA Therapy Approaches

Let me hear your voice: A family's triumph over autism by Catherine Maurice

Teaching developmentally disabled children: The me book by O. Ivar Lovaas

Behavioral intervention for young children with autism: A manual for parents and professionals by Catherine Maurice, Gina Green, and Stephen C. Luce

Right from the start: Behavioral intervention for young children with autism, second edition (Topics in autism), by Sandra L. Harris and Mary Jane Weiss

Functional behavior assessment for people with autism: Making sense of seemingly senseless behavior (topics in autism) authored by Beth A. Glasberg

The verbal behavior approach: How to teach children with autism and related disorders by Mary Barbera and Tracy Rasmussen

Pivotal response treatments for autism: Communication, social, & academic development by Robert L. Koegel and Lynn Kern Koegel

Overcoming autism: Finding the answers, strategies, and hope that can transform a child's life by Lynn Kern Koegel and Claire LaZebnik

Self-help skills for people with autism: A systematic teaching approach (topics in autism) by Stephen R. Anderson, Amy L. Jablonski, Vicki Madaus Knapp, and Marcus L. Thomeer

Sense and nonsense in the behavioral treatment of autism: It has to be said by Ron Leaf, John McEachin, and Mitch Taubman

It's time for school!: Building quality ABA educational programs for students with autism spectrum disorders by Ronald Leaf, Mitchell Taubman, and John McEachin

A work in progress: Behavior management strategies & a curriculum for intensive behavioral treatment of autism by Ronald Leaf, John McEachin, and Jaisom D. Harsh

Teaching conversation to children with autism: Scripts and script fading (topics in autism) by Lynn E. McClannahan and Patricia J. Krantz

Activity schedules for children with autism by Lynn E. McClannahan and Patricia J. Krantz

Behavior/speak: A glossary of terms in applied behavior analysis by
Bobby Newman, Kenneth F. Reeve, Sharon A. Reeve, and Carolyn
S. Ryan

*Teaching children with autism: Strategies for initiating positive
interactions and improving learning opportunities* by Robert L.
Koegel and Lynn Kern Koegel

Web Sites and Material on ABA and Autism

http://rsaffran.tripod.com/whatisaba.html

This web site gives a brief description of ABA, Discrete trial training, and helpful links to other sites. Click on ABA resources and there
is a wealth of information.

http://www.eparent.com

This is the web site for *Exceptional Parent* magazine a monthly pub-
lication that provides information for parents, teachers, clinicians, and
advocates with an interest in autism and other developmental disabilities.

Videos for *ABA therapy and autism*

This caption can be found by placing into a search engine (I used
Google) the following: ABA therapy and autism. Here you will see captured videos of ABA teaching and therapy sequences of children with
autism.

http://health.yahoo.com/nervous-videos/aba-therapy-for-autism/healthi-
nation-HNB10081_autism_4.html

This is a short video that highlights a discussion of ABA with
Dr. Doreen Granpeesheh, Ph.D., and the services her agency provides. She
is the founder of the Center for Autism and Related Disorders (CARD).

ABA Web Sites

www.bacb.com

This site is the official site for the Behavior Analysis Certification
Board. It provides a directory of people who are Board Certified
Behavior Analyst (BCBA) having met requirements for certification to
practice behavior analysis. Click on "Maintain Certification" and you
will see a link to a certificant registry, which you can click on to get to
the directory of certified people. You can select how many miles from

your area you want to search and a list of names and their distance from you is provided. You can e-mail them from this site.

Also, there is a link to university-approved programs that provide the coursework that is approved by the Board to meet the criteria required to take the national boards. The coordinator of these university programs could also provide a resource for ABA technical assistance and direct service for your family. You will click on the country you reside in, and then if United States, click on the state and you will see stars that identify universities where their graduate program is approved by the Behavior Analyst Certification Board to offer courses that can lead to qualifying to take the national board certification test.

www.abainternational.org

This site is sponsored by the international association for ABA.

www.fabaworld.org

This is the site for the Florida ABA, where the certification for behavior analysts was born in the 1980s. There is a wealth of information about ABA.

http://www.dds.ca.gov/rc/rclist.cfm

In California, services for persons with disabilities are provided through Regional Centers, and this site lists the Regional Centers and the counties they serve. You can also use a search engine on the Internet to obtain clinics with diagnostic, assessment, and intervention services for children with ASD and their families.

Autism Advocacy and Support Groups

www.**autism**speaks.org

www.**autisticadvocacy**.org

www.national**autism**association.org

www.parentsofchildrenwith**autism**.org/**autism_advocacy_groups**.htm

www.**autism**-society.org

www.autcom.org

www.childrensdisabilities.info/autism/groups-autism-asperger.html

This site provides an annotated list of *support groups* and listservs for *parents* of children with *Autism*, Asperger's Syndrome, or Pervasive Developmental Delay.

Index